600 MCQs in Anaesthesia: Basic Sciences

600 MCQs in Anaesthesia: Basic Sciences

Neville W. Goodman
MA DPhil FRCA

Consultant Senior Lecturer in Anaesthesia, University of Bristol and Southmead Hospital, Bristol, UK

Chris Johnson
MA MD FRCA

Consultant Anaesthetist, Southmead Hospital and Clinical Lecturer, University of Bristol, Bristol, UK

SECOND EDITION

Churchill Livingstone 🏛

EDINBURGH LONDON MADRID MELBOURNE NEW YORK AND TOKYO 1994

CHURCHILL LIVINGSTONE
Medical Division of Longman Group UK Limited

Distributed in the United States of America by Churchill
Livingstone Inc., 650 Avenue of the Americas, New York, N.Y.
10011, and by associated companies, branches and
representatives throughout the world.

First edition 1985
Second edition 1994

ISBN 0 443 04831 2

British Library Cataloguing in Publication Data
A catalogue record for this book is available from the British
Library.

Library of Congress Cataloging in Publication Data
Goodman, N. W.
    600 MCQs in anaesthesia : basic sciences / Neville W. Goodman,
Chris Johnson. — 2nd ed.
        p.   cm.
    Includes Index.
    Rev. ed. of: 600 MCQs in anaesthesia / P.J. Simpson, N.W. Goodman.
1985.
    ISBN 0–443–04831–2
    1. Anesthesiology—Examinations, questions, etc. 2. Medical
sciences—Examinations, questions, etc.   I. Johnson, Chris,
FRCAnaes. II. Simpson, Peter J.   600 MCQ in anesthesia.
III. Title.   IV. Title: Six hundred MCQs in anaesthesia.
    [DNLM: 1. Anesthesiology— examination questions.   2. Science—
—examination questions.   WO 218 G653z   1993]
RD 82.3.S48   1993
617.9'6'076—dc20
DNLM/DLC
for Library of Congress   93–12699

Produced by Longman Singapore Publishers Pte Ltd
Printed in Singapore

Contents

Preface

This is the second edition of a book that provides examination practice at multiple choice questions on the basic sciences for the diploma of Fellow of the Royal College of Anaesthetists (FRCA). The questions are arranged in mock papers of 30 MCQs, to allow candidates to time themselves answering questions similar to those they will encounter in the actual examination, and each paper is followed by annotated answers. The book will help with the need to get a feel for MCQ papers before being faced with the real thing in the examination hall.

Although aimed at the Part 2 FRCA, many of the simpler topics are relevant to Part 1, and the book will provide revision for Part 3. Candidates for the European Diploma of Anaesthesiology should also benefit.

Unlike those books of MCQs arranged under topic headings, candidates will have to be adaptable, not only to the topic changing from question to question, but also to the degree of difficulty – and, as is bound to happen in the actual examination, candidates will find some questions that they cannot answer.

There are few questions in this second edition that are exactly the same as in the first edition. About 15% of the questions are entirely new, bringing the book up to date. Many of the others have had one or two branches replaced, and most have had the wording altered to make the questions clearer. The answers to many questions have been expanded.

Some alterations for this second edition came after trainee anaesthetists in Bristol pointed out errors in the first edition and we thank them. We are not afraid to receive similar comments about this edition, but remind candidates that in the actual examination they will never know what the examiners' answers were. If this book allows candidates to identify gaps in their knowledge before the examination, or if it encourages discussion between candidates and tutors about what is a correct answer, then it will have served its purpose.

Bristol, 1994

N. G.
C. J.

Introduction to the second edition

Since the first edition, the new examination structure has become established. The clinical examinations of Part 1 and Part 3 are separated by the basic science examination of Part 2. This book is aimed at Part 2. Parts 1 and 3 do examine all the sciences as they relate to clinical practice but, with Part 2 now formally consisting of the two parts physiology and pharmacology, there is without doubt less examination of physics than there used to be.

We have modified the structure of the first edition, in which 10 'papers' of 60 mixed questions were to be each answered in sittings of 1¾ hours. Recognising that 1¾ hours is a long time to put aside for undisturbed study, there are now 20 'papers' of 30 mixed questions, each paper to be answered in 45 minutes. The 'Physics and clinical measurement' of the first edition has become simply 'Clinical measurement', and there are fewer questions on true physics. Replaced questions in this section have been substituted by questions on physiological measurement and on the use of the monitoring devices that are now in more common use than in 1985.

The nature of progress in anaesthetic science means that there are more new questions in pharmacology than in physiology; new drugs appear and their actions and side-effects have to be understood, but the principles of physiology change little. Certainly the details of physiology are becoming more complex as they become more understood but, to return to 'The last word' of the introduction to the first edition, that generates more trees but obscures the wood.

Because of these changes since the first edition, each paper is no longer strictly one-third physiology, one-third pharmacology and one-third clinical measurement. Although the exact proportion varies, about 24 of each 30 questions are physiology and pharmacology, leaving 6 for measurement, of which some are heavily physiological.

There are few questions that are precisely as they were in the first edition. MCQs are better if stem and branches are always complete sentences, so we have altered those that were not. We have simplified many questions and, we think, made them easier. Practice questions should not be easier than those in the examination, but candidates did say after the first edition that some were perhaps too testing – and too discouraging. Many answers are now given more fully. Readers are invited to write to the authors if they find an incorrect answer, though we have tried to check them all. But bear in mind that of greatest importance is your overall score on a paper; and that in the examination hall you will never know what the examiners think is the correct answer.

Introduction

There are two things that you must do to pass the examinations for the diploma of the FRCA: you must reach a certain level of knowledge; and you must know how to present it to the examiners. This is the first of two books that are more concerned with the second of these requirements; they will also help you to assess your level of knowledge, but they should not be treated as sources of knowledge.

The standard textbooks are the best source books of basic knowledge for the FRCA. The more specialised texts, reviews in the journals, and discussion with others should be used to build upon this knowledge – to update it and to find faults in it. You cannot expect to pass an examination unless you work for it: the more clinically oriented the examination, the more importance you must place on gaining wide experience in clinical anaesthesia. You must avoid the danger of working too much 'at the books'.

Many people think that the key to these exams is to go on a course, and there is no doubt that courses can be extremely useful. They should, however, be thought of as a means of aiming one's studies in the right directions; it is disappointing to find that many people will attend a course 2–3 months before the hurdle of a major examination apparently without previously having done any work. This is foolhardy. To get the most out of a course, one should have covered some of the groundwork beforehand. Once you have acquired what you hope to be sufficient knowledge (and in the absence of a published syllabus this must be a matter of guesswork in some areas), then is the time that these books should be of help to you.

How to answer multiple choice questions

The format of the MCQs in the FRCA examination is a stem and five branches. The stem may be short ('Opiates are:'), or may be a few lines, for example when presenting a clinical problem. Each of the five branches that follow may be true or false. You score one mark for each correct answer, minus one for each incorrect answer, and, extremely important to the examination technique, you score nothing if you choose not to answer a particular branch. Your actual answers are marked by computer, and so you must eventually put your answers on to special cards that are supplied separately. These cards have the question numbers printed on them and you indicate your answer by filling in a 'true' or a 'false' box in pencil.

The most important tactic is not to guess: if you don't know – leave that branch blank. You should also think very carefully if you think a branch (or a stem) is ambiguous.

You must read each stem very carefully: watch out for qualifying words such as 'commonly', 'rarely', 'always' and the like because they can turn what would otherwise be a 'false' into a 'true' and vice versa. Re-read the stem with each statement: it is all too easy to forget the emphasis and exact wording of the stem as you work down the five branches. Watch out for negatives: in the heat of the moment you may fail to see 'not' in a branch. 'May' is an awkward word; one can argue that anything 'may' cause anything else. Try to give the answer relevant to clinical practice: for instance, it is 'true' that atropine may cause bradycardia, but not that propranolol may relieve bronchospasm.

There are some subjects on which questions tend to be particularly confusing: the oxyhaemoglobin dissociation curve is one, the ionic dissociation of drugs is another. These are both subjects in which the wording of stem and branch are crucial. If an option states 'The saturated vapour pressure of halothane is 243 mmHg', then the answer is clear (if you happen to know!); but the concept and consequences of 'The oxyhaemoglobin dissociation curve is shifted to the left by hypercarbia' can be expressed in a number of different ways – and even then the wording of the stem may alter the answer. When we think that a question is of this type we make a comment about it which you can read along with the answer: we try to point out how a question is confusing.

It is impossible to write an MCQ paper without some of them being ambiguous – or seeming ambiguous to some people. Some of our questions may be ambiguous and we apologise for this, but some of the questions in the actual examination paper will be ambiguous, or will seem so to you in the examination hall, and you must learn how to deal with them.

It is often more difficult to think of false branches than true branches when compiling MCQ questions. Questions tend to fall into two basic types: the straightforward factual type and the deductive type. Many pharmacology questions present facts: a drug and five properties that may or may not be properties of that drug. A false branch must appear to some candidates to be true or else the question will not discriminate between the good and poor candidate. The false branches are likely to be: the exact opposite of the true answer (for example, hyperkalaemia for hypokalaemia), an association with another similar or similar-sounding drug (for example, a property of chlorpropamide appended to a question on chlorpromazine), or a complete red herring. These last can be very difficult to answer, and you may not be able to find the correct answer in the literature because the connection does not exist. False answers in the deductive type of question include these types, although they may not be so obvious, but also include answers of false logic.

A strategy for a multiple choice paper

You should have a general strategy for answering an MCQ paper. For those who haven't, we suggest one here. We are not saying it is the only one, but we think it allows efficient use of the time spent answering the paper.

First, read through the questions from the first to the last answering quickly those of which you are certain of the answers. Mark the options T or F on the question paper; it is not a good idea to mark the computer card as you go because it is then not as easy to check your answers.

You will probably find that you can tell from the stem whether or not you will be able to answer a question. If you cannot answer a question immediately on this first read-through, put a question mark by it if you will need to think about it (and by any answers that you do make of which you are a little uncertain), and put a cross against those that you think you will probably not be able to answer at all. It is very important not to dwell on doubtful questions at all first time through or you may find yourself short of time before you have answered all the questions that you do know.

On the second read-through, tackle those that you marked with a question mark; don't be afraid to scribble formulas or graphs on scrap paper to help you with confusing questions. After this second read-through it is worth going back and rechecking the answers – but don't dwell on those that you answered on the first read-through or you will find yourself doubting even your most cast-iron certainties. At this stage, transfer the answers that you have made so far to the computer cards and *make sure that you mark the cards correctly*; it is easy to get out of phase between the question numbers and answer numbers. You should now regard these answers as immutable: don't look at the questions again and get on with answering those that you marked with a cross. Answers to these questions you can transfer to the computer cards right away because you will have had plenty of time to think around the subject.

When you have answered all you can, check that you have written your name everywhere that you should have done, and it may be better to leave the examination hall. With essay questions, you should always be able to add more to your answers and you should stay for every precious minute; staying and staring at MCQ answers induces neurosis.

The MCQ papers in this book

The 600 questions are arranged in 20 'papers' of 30 questions. a 'paper' consists of 10–12 questions on each of physiology and pharmacology, clinical measurement making up the rest. The present format of the MCQ paper in the Part 2 examination is 80 questions in 2¾ hours and we suggest that the best way to test yourself is to try a whole 'paper' *under examination conditions, unseen, in 45 minutes.* If you take longer than this you may run out of time in the examination when transferring your answers to the computer cards. The index at the back of the book allows you to find questions under broad subject headings so that you could, if you wanted, answer a number of questions from different papers on, say, endocrine physiology. You will, however, gain nothing if you look at the answers without trying the questions; and there is little to gain from trying a question if you have not done the work on the subject. There are more questions on some topics than on others. Some of the questions in the later papers on these important topics are similar to the questions in earlier papers and will allow you to assess whether your factual recall or your understanding of the topic has improved.

How to score yourself

For each branch, score + 1 if you marked correctly TRUE or FALSE, or – 1 if you marked incorrectly TRUE or FALSE. Score 0 for any branch for which you gave no answer. The maximum for each question is thus + 5, and the minimum is – 5.

Your overall score on a 'paper' will give some idea of your general level of knowledge. We cannot say what score corresponds to a 'pass' in the MCQ in the actual examination, but, from our experience of setting mock papers to candidates in the past, you should be looking for 50% at the very least (75/150) for one 'paper', and 70% (105/150) is a good score.

As well as your overall score it is worth calculating your 'efficiency ratio', which is your number of correct answers expressed as a percentage of your total number of attempted answers. Thus you can get an overall score of 50% by answering 75 branches correctly (an efficiency of 100%) or by answering 95 but getting 10 of them wrong: 85 × (+ 1) minus 10 × (– 1). A low total score with a high efficiency implies that you are certain of what you know but your overall knowledge is not enough; a low efficiency ratio means that your knowledge is faulty, or that you are guessing.

Often, candidates going up for the examination ask how many branches they should aim to answer. The only sensible answer to this is that you should answer all that you can. There is no 'safe' number. Certainly, if you are able to answer only 40%, then that is unlikely to be enough to pass, but merely ploughing on and guessing to bring your total answered up above 50% is unlikely to increase your score because half of your additional answers, if they are pure guesses, will be incorrect. Similarly, if you have answered 60%, don't assume that there is no need to answer any more – you may have answered incorrectly more than you think.

Your overall score will indicate your knowledge; your efficiency ratio will point out gross faults in technique of answering; you should also look very carefully at those individual questions at which you scored badly. Using the same reasoning as for the complete paper, you will need to score 3 out of 5 to 'pass' a single question. Think carefully why you did poorly on a particular question. The usual reason is simply lack of knowledge and occasionally you will find a complete gap such that you are unable to answer any of the branches of a question. A very high negative score (– 4 or – 5) usually implies a lack of understanding of the question rather than lack of knowledge, or a misunderstanding or misreading of the wording. These high negative scores have a great effect on your overall score and perhaps one of the main lessons of this book is to help you to avoid them. As we have stressed before, it is essential *to read each question very carefully*: don't rush at the questions.

The answers and comments

In the answer section for each paper we give explanations of the correct answers and also make comments, if appropriate, on the form and wording of the question. It is very easy to become side-tracked and obsessed when you get a particular branch wrong which you feel you marked correctly. You may find a source which shows you are indeed correct. However, nobody fails the MCQ paper because of one branch that, according to the 'correct' answer, they answered incorrectly; concentrate instead on those questions on which you did badly overall. If you scored – 3 on a question about acid-base balance it would be more valuable to go and read a good account of acid-base balance and to seek help from others than to feel aggrieved that you think we are wrong on one particular point and waste time laboriously checking each particular branch.

We cannot give full explanations for all the branches in all the questions: that would mean writing a large textbook. Some questions demand more explanation than others and some questions have very short comments. For many of the more important topics we advise you to consult the textbooks if you do badly. There are no references quoted, but it should be possible to answer all the questions in the book from reading of the standard texts.

The last word

The examiners try to set clear and unambiguous questions on sensible, mainstream subjects. They are not trying to be devious and trick you into giving incorrect answers. It is often said that MCQs are unfair because they penalise candidates who have read widely and who can always find a reason why 'true' is actually 'sometimes true' or 'may be true', but MCQs have to have black-or-white answers. When testing basic knowledge or general principles what the examiner wants to know is whether the candidate can see the wood for the trees.

Paper I Questions

I.1   **The following are intracellular buffers:**
- **A**   bicarbonate and carbonic acid
- **B**   hydroxyapatite
- **C**   albumin
- **D**   inorganic phosphate
- **E**   haemoglobin.

I.2   **These are essential amino acids:**
- **A**   methionine
- **B**   glycine
- **C**   leucine
- **D**   tyrosine
- **E**   alanine.

I.3   **In the electrocardiogram at a heart rate of 80 per minute:**
- **A**   the PR interval should be less than 0.2 s and greater than 0.12 s
- **B**   the QRS complex should last less than 0.02 s
- **C**   the T wave is normally greater than 1 mV
- **D**   there will be an interval of 0.75 s between the end of one complex and the beginning of the next
- **E**   the T wave is ventricular repolarisation.

I.4   **When the nerve cell membrane is suddenly depolarised:**
- **A**   sodium conductance rapidly increases
- **B**   potassium conductance rapidly increases
- **C**   the membrane potential becomes zero
- **D**   intracellular sodium concentration rises very little
- **E**   the sodium/potassium ATPase pump is activated.

I.5   **One or more prostaglandins:**
- **A**   are peptide hormones
- **B**   dilate the bronchi
- **C**   stimulate uterine contractions
- **D**   increase the intracranial pressure
- **E**   affect platelet function.

I.6   In the control of body temperature:
A   shivering is a spinal reflex
B   energy from brown fat is released by sympathetic stimulation
C   brain amines are important
D   at an environmental temperature of 21°C most heat loss is by vaporisation of sweat
E   control is independent of higher centres.

I.7   Fibrinogen degradation products are natural anticoagulants interfering with:
A   polymerisation of the fibrin monomer
B   platelet aggregation
C   thrombin activity
D   serum calcium concentrations
E   intrinsic pathway activation.

I.8   After drinking one litre of one-tenth molar ammonium chloride solution:
A   the urine will become acid
B   urine output will fall
C   the plasma bicarbonate will fall
D   the subject will become extremely thirsty
E   the ammonium ions will be converted to urea.

I.9   The following are true of the renal circulation:
A   reduction from systemic arterial pressure is chiefly at the efferent glomerular arterioles
B   renal vasoconstriction is stimulated by a decreased baroreceptor discharge
C   a 50% reduction in arterial PO_2 produces a significant reduction in renal blood flow
D   renal vasodilation is a dopaminergic response
E   glomerular perfusion pressure is controlled by local autoregulatory mechanisms.

I.10   Under normal circumstances, the following statements about blood gases are true:
A   the normal venous PO_2 is approximately 5.2 kPa (40 mmHg)
B   the normal venous oxygen saturation is 75%
C   2.0 ml oxygen is dissolved in 100 ml blood
D   nitrogen is only carried in arterial blood in the dissolved form
E   there is approximately 49 ml CO_2 combined with haemoglobin in 100 ml of arterial blood.

I.11 Stagnant hypoxia occurs in:

A pulmonary fibrosis
B myocardial infarction
C massive haemorrhage
D carbon monoxide poisoning
E hypothermia.

I.12 The following antibiotics are actively secreted by the kidneys:

A benzyl penicillin
B tetracycline
C chloramphenicol
D neomycin
E cefuroxime.

I.13 Atropine:

A has no effect on acetylcholine production or destruction
B dilates cutaneous blood vessels
C is a parasympathetic depressant
D stimulates the respiratory centre
E increases intraocular pressure.

I.14 Drugs which exert an autonomic ganglion blocking effect include:

A decamethonium
B barbiturates
C atropine
D trimetaphan
E phentolamine.

I.15 The following are aldosterone antagonists:

A triamterene
B spironolactone
C digoxin
D dopamine
E diazoxide.

I.16 Metyrapone:

A is used therapeutically in Cushing's syndrome
B inhibits the production of both cortisol and aldosterone
C causes increased corticotrophin levels
D must be given intravenously
E response is measured by analysing urinary steroids

I.17 Etomidate:

A may cause an epileptic fit
B is metabolised by Hoffman elimination
C may produce immunologically-mediated hypersensitivity reactions
D possesses analgesic properties
E is soluble in water.

I.18 Thiopentone:

A is 50–75% bound to plasma proteins at normal plasma pH
B is a thiosubstituted succinylurea
C in the standard 2.5% solution has a pH greater than 9
D after re-distribution is rapidly metabolised in the liver
E excretion is usefully accelerated by a forced alkaline diuresis.

I.19 Insulin:

A increases formation of both liver and muscle glycogen
B inhibits gluconeogenesis
C reduces protein synthesis
D decreases serum potassium
E increases fat synthesis.

I.20 Pseudocholinesterase:

A is found in plasma
B is inhibited by organophosphorus compounds
C plasma concentrations are reduced during pregnancy
D is stimulated by fluoride ions
E is responsible for the inactivation of succinylcholine.

I.21 Pentazocine:

A produces less respiratory depression than that induced by an equianalgesic dose of morphine
B is a weak agonist at μ-receptors
C induces respiratory depression reversible by naloxone
D will reverse respiratory depression caused by fentanyl
E induces confusion in the elderly.

I.22 A plot of pressure against volume:

A allows compliance to be measured
B shows hysteresis
C allows a direct measurement of airways resistance
D is usually plotted on semi-logarithmic paper
E allows an estimate to be made of respiratory work.

I.23 Clinical trials:

A   are 'single-blind' when only the subject is unaware of the treatment used
B   are 'double-blind' when neither investigators nor subjects are aware of the treatment used
C   if single-blind do not require placebo control
D   if double-blind are unsuitable for sequential analysis
E   if double-blind do not prevent observer bias.

I.24 Soda lime:

A   contains 90% sodium hydroxide with 5% potassium hydroxide
B   must be moist to function
C   has an exothermic reaction with carbon dioxide
D   becomes exhausted more rapidly with high fresh gas flows
E   reduces atmospheric pollution by anaesthetic vapours.

I.25 The following are true of vaporisers and anaesthetic circuits:

A   with the vaporiser inside a circle (VIC), the inflow gas contains an unknown concentration of volatile agent
B   with VIC, an efficient vaporiser is needed to maintain an accurate vapour concentration within the circuit
C   with the vaporiser outside the circle (VOC), an inefficient vaporiser is satisfactory because inspired concentrations are not critical
D   with VOC, the anaesthetic vapour concentration within the circuit is dependent upon uptake by the patient
E   with VIC and low fresh gas flow, the inspired concentration is greater than the vaporiser setting.

I.26 There are electromanometers which work on the principle of:

A   the fuel cell
B   variable capacitance
C   variable inductance
D   the Wheatstone bridge
E   variable conductance.

I.27 The following statements about gauges and sizes are true:

A   a catheter of 28FG will have a circumference of 28 mm
B   a needle of 21SWG is smaller than one of 23SWG
C   a short cannula of 14SWG external diameter will allow a maximum flow of one litre in about 4 min
D   an endotracheal tube size 8 will have an external diameter of 8 mm
E   the standard BS tapers are 15, 22 and 32 mm.

I.28 The following are inflammable:

A   ethyl chloride
B   0.5% chlorhexidine in 70% alcohol
C   cyclopropane in oxygen
D   nitrous oxide at high temperatures
E   diethyl ether.

I.29 In the Astrup interpolation method of blood gas analysis:

A   the buffer line for a particular blood sample is obtained by tonometry with two different carbon dioxide concentrations
B   the only direct measurement is of pH
C   buffer base can be derived by plotting pH against PCO_2 on a Siggaard–Anderson nomogram
D   plasma protein concentration must be known
E   phosphate buffers of standard pH are used for spanning the pH electrode.

I.30 The following are true of surface tension:

A   it is measured in newtons per square metre
B   it acts vertically and horizontally at the junction between a fluid and the wall of a containing vessel
C   the pressure generated by surface tension in a sphere is double that in a tube
D   the transmural pressure of a sphere is directly proportional to the radius of the sphere
E   surface tension is a direct result of molecular attraction at the surface of the liquid.

Paper I Answers

I.1   TTFFT

A   The bicarbonate system is much more important as an extracellular buffer, but the answer is still 'true'.
B   Hydroxyapatite is an intracellular buffer in bone.
C   Albumin is an *extracellular* buffer.
D   *Organic* phosphates are intracellular buffers.
E   Haemoglobin is a buffer because of the imidazole groups of the histidine residues.

I.2   TFTFF

D   Tyrosine is non-essential unless phenylalanine is missing from the diet.

I.3   TFFFT

B   The QRS complex is up to 0.1 s.
C   The amplitude of the QRS is usually 1–2 mV; the amplitude of the T wave is much less.
D   The *R–R interval* will be 0.75 s.

I.4   TFFTF

B   The increase is relatively slow and restores resting potential.
C   There is a positive transmembrane potential.
D   The shift in ions per action potential is less than 1/100 000 of the total ions in the cell.
E   The sodium/potassium ATPase works continuously.

I.5   FTTFT

A   The prostaglandins are unsaturated fatty acids (not peptides).
B   They have a great variety of actions in many tissues and it would be unproductive to try and learn them all.
C,E They are now used clinically (for example, for their effects on the uterus, on platelets, and to prevent closure of the ductus). You ought to know clinically useful actions.
D   Injection of prostaglandins into the IIIrd ventricle may cause fever but not an increase in intracranial pressure.

I.6   FTTFF

    A   Shivering depends on central coordination.

    B   There are sympathetically innervated deposits of brown fat in children and adults.

    C   There are species differences; 5-hydroxytryptamine and noradrenaline have been implicated.

    D   At 21°C 70% of heat loss is by radiation and conduction.

    E   Temperature causes changes in behaviour, for example, decreased activity on a very hot day.

I.7   TTTFF

    D,E   There is no evidence that fibrinogen degradation products interfere with either of these mechanisms.

I.8   TFTFT

    A   Ammonium chloride is an acidifying salt used, in suitable combination with other electrolyte solutions, in severe metabolic alkalosis.

    B   It is a diuretic, increasing urine output by supplying an acid load.

    D   The diuresis is not dramatic, and ammonium chloride has no specific property of inducing thirst.

    E   Conversion of ammonium to urea occurs in the liver.

I.9   TTTTF

    E   Local mechanisms are not involved. Alterations in renal perfusion occur in response to systemic effects.

I.10   TTFTF

    C   The normal figure for dissolved oxygen is 0.3 ml/dl.

    E   The figure is correct but for the *total* CO_2 in the blood not the amount combined with haemoglobin. Of the 49 ml/dl, 2.6 ml is dissolved, 2.6 ml is combined as carbamino compounds and 43.8 ml is in the form of bicarbonate ions.

I.11 FTFFT

Stagnant hypoxia is caused by a slow circulation in certain conditions of shock.
A   Pulmonary fibrosis causes hypoxic hypoxia.
B   Myocardial infarction causing cardiogenic shock will cause stagnant hypoxia.
C   Haemorrhage is anaemic hypoxia.
E   Peripheral stagnation is common in hypothermia.

I.12 TFTFT

C   A question of small print. Unaltered chloramphenicol is excreted by glomerular filtration, but the inactive degradation products are secreted by the tubules.

I.13 TTTTT

D   Atropine is a general central stimulant.
E   Atropine increases intraocular pressure by mydriasis but, at least with normal clinical doses, only when applied topically.

I.14 TTTTF

A   Decamethonium (now of historical importance only) has a similar structure to acetylcholine.
B,C Barbiturates probably act on preganglionic nerve endings, changing properties necessary for normal transmission.
D   Trimetaphan is a competitive ganglion blocker.
E   Phentolamine is an α-adrenergic blocker.

I.15 TTFFF

C   The diuretic effect of digoxin is secondary to increased renal perfusion.
D   The diuretic action of dopamine is via its effect on cardiac output and its specific dopaminergic renal effect.
E   Diazoxide is not a diuretic.

I.16 TTTFT

Metyrapone is a competitive inhibitor of 11β-hydroxylation in the synthesis of steroids and is used in the diagnosis of adrenocorticoid disorders.
A   True: though mainly diagnostic, it can also be used therapeutically if other treatments are not practical.
C   The feedback loop is broken.
D   Metyrapone can be given orally.

I.17   FFFFF

A   Etomidate causes involuntary movements but is not epileptogenic.

B   Atracurium is metabolised by Hoffman elimination.

C   There have been documented reactions due to direct histamine release but they are rare.

E   Etomidate is solubilised, in the current formulation, in propylene glycol.

I.18   TFTFF

B   Malonyl urea.

D   Metabolised, but only at 10–15% per hour.

E   Its excretion is speeded by alkaline urine, but not 'usefully'.

I.19   TTFTT

B   True: insulin inhibits gluconeogenesis and ketogenesis.

C   Insulin *increases* protein synthesis.

I.20   TTTFT

B   'Organophosphorus compounds' include insecticides and 'nerve gases'. Their main action is on acetylcholinesterase but they also inactivate other esterases.

D   Fluoride is a differential inhibitor, used in the diagnosis of atypical enzyme.

I.21   FTFTT

A   Analgesic effect equates with respiratory depression for most opioids.

B   Pentazocine is an agonist at κ-receptors, but a weak antagonist at μ-receptors.

C   The respiratory depression of pentazocine is only reversible in a non-specific way, by analeptic drugs such as doxapram.

D   True: this has been used as a technique for postoperative analgesia.

I.22   TTFFT

B   True: the relation between pressure and volume is different when the pressure is increasing from when it is decreasing. The plot shows a 'hysteresis loop'.

C   Resistance implies flow, which is volume per *time*. Neither pressure nor volume includes a consideration of time.

E   Work is force multiplied by distance. The application of simple algebra and your knowledge of the meaning of pressure and volume should show that work is pressure multiplied by volume.

I.23   TTFFT

C   The degree of blindness does not affect the need for a placebo.

D   Sequential analysis is simply a way of comparing two alternatives and is suitable for a double-blind study. ✓

E   Bias covers more than just the bias toward one group or the other; it refers also to, for example, the bias towards recording blood pressures that are not too low.

I.24   FTTFF

A   This would be highly caustic; soda lime contains 90% calcium hydroxide, with 5% sodium hydroxide, 1% potassium hydroxide and some silicates.

D   The rate of exhaustion depends upon the carbon dioxide production of the patients.

E   Not by itself, although it does allow lower fresh gas flows and thus avoids waste and pollution indirectly.

I.25   FFFTT

This question is not difficult, but may need a bit of thought.

A   False. With VIC the inflow gas (FGF) contains no volatile agent.

B   False – an inefficient vaporiser (for example, Goldman's) should be used otherwise vapour concentrations will rapidly become high. Monitoring of vapour concentration is a good idea if this system is used.

C   False. With VOC there is low inflow, so this gas must be able to contain high concentrations of volatile agent.

E   True. Expired volatile agent is recycled.

I.26   FTTTT

An electromanometer can be based on many electrical components.

A   The fuel cell is the basis for a method of measuring oxygen.

D   A Wheatstone bridge is a circuit of resistances that can be balanced for nil current flow.

I.27   TFTFF

A   FG is French gauge: the number depends upon circumference and a larger number means a bigger catheter.

B   In Steel Wire Gauge the number is the number of wires that will fit in a standard hole: the larger the number, the smaller the wire.

C   The flow depends on the internal, not the external, diameter. Nonetheless, this is a realistic figure for such a cannula (actually the quoted rate from a 14G Venflon®).

D   Endotracheal tubes are measured by *internal* diameter. The external diameter may be marked on disposable tubes.

E   These are the tapers on anaesthetic circuits: 15 and 22 are correct, but the exhaust taper is 30 mm.

I.28   TTTFT

A   True. Squirting this stuff around (to test sensory levels, for example) can be dangerous, especially as it pools.

B   True. An important source of fires and burns is pools of spirit solutions under the operative drapes.

C,E   True. Of historical interest only now, but the reason why much money was spent on antistatic precautions.

D   False. Nitrous oxide is neither flammable nor explosive but it supports combustion at temperatures above 450°C, when it starts to break down to nitrogen and oxygen.

I.29   TTTFT

Although not used now, the Astrup method is the basis of current methods of blood gas analysis, and is often asked about.

B   True: using a pH glass electrode.

D   In clinical practice the variations of plasma proteins affect the buffering power of blood little, but haemoglobin has considerable buffering power and its concentration must be known.

I.30   FTTFT

A   Surface tension is force per unit length: newtons per metre.

D   From Laplace's law, the transmural pressure of a sphere is directly proportional to the surface tension of the liquid and indirectly proportional to the radius of the sphere.

Paper II Questions

II.1 **The following statements about autonomic ganglia are true:**

A the main neurotransmitter is noradrenaline
B parasympathetic ganglia are situated close to target organs
C they are linked to the spinal cord by grey rami communicantes
D they relay preganglionic to postganglionic impulses
E removal of both lumbar sympathetic chains is fatal.

II.2 **In the cardiac cycle:**

A left ventricular volume is maximal at the end of atrial systole
B the mitral valve closes by contraction of the papillary muscles
C the left ventricular pressure is maximal just before the aortic valve opens
D the ejection fraction is about 85%
E the dicrotic notch is due to rebound of the aortic valve.

II.3 **Pulmonary vascular resistance:**

A is increased in chronic hypoxia
B has a value approximately one-sixth that of the systemic circulation
C can be measured using a flow-directed balloon catheter with a thermistor tip
D is increased by isoprenaline
E is decreased by 5-hydroxytryptamine (5-HT).

II.4   The following are true of sensory receptors:

A   receptor adaptation implies a decline in frequency of receptor discharge after onset of a steady stimulus

B   cutaneous sensory receptors respond to several sensory modalities

C   the sensation evoked by a receptor is determined by the part of brain it innervates

D   proprioceptors each only respond to a specific stimulus

E   stretch receptors are rapidly-adapting.

II.5   The pituitary gland responds to secretions from the:

A   hypothalamus

B   adrenal medulla

C   adrenal cortex

D   pancreas

E   thyroid.

II.6   The following are true of peristalsis in the small intestine:

A   it depends on an intact parasympathetic nervous system

B   it is coordinated by a slow wave of depolarisation

C   stretch initiates the myenteric reflex

D   vasoactive intestinal peptide (VIP) is a potent inhibitor

E   it is inhibited by sympathetic discharge in the splanchnic nerves.

II.7   The following are true of pancreatic exocrine secretion:

A   insulin is secreted in response to an increase in blood glucose

B   cholecystokinin (CCK) stimulates an enzyme-rich secretion

C   secretion is not influenced by the vagus

D   atropine blocks the effects of secretin and cholecystokinin

E   it contains a trypsin inhibitor.

II.8   Compared with extracellular fluid, the intracellular fluid contains a greater concentration of:

A   sodium ions

B   magnesium ions

C   protein

D   hydrogen ions

E   bicarbonate ions.

Na 145 : 12

Na   Mg 2 : 15

Poten 15 : 60

bic   pH 7.4 : 7.0

bicab 27 : 8

II.9   In the control of respiration:

  A   hypoxic drive originates in the peripheral chemoreceptors
  B   there is no measurable hypoxic drive in a normal subject
      breathing air at sea level
  C   the response to CO_2 is linear over the normal range
  D   the increased drive in exercise is due to incomplete oxygen
      equilibration in the pulmonary capillaries
  E   the gasping respiration of shock is a baroreceptor reflex.

II.10   The following proportions of haemoglobin may be found in
        the arterial blood of a normal adult breathing room air:

  A   5–10% carboxyhaemoglobin
  B   4% methaemoglobin
  C   2% free haemoglobin
  D   2% fetal haemoglobin
  E   25% reduced haemoglobin.

II.11   The effect of hypercapnia upon the oxyhaemoglobin
        dissociation curve is:

  A   to shift the curve to the left
  B   to reduce the affinity of haemoglobin for oxygen
  C   dependent on body temperature
  D   masked by decreases in 2,3-DPG
  E   enhanced in anaemia.

II.12   Dopamine:

  A   increases cardiac output
  B   in high doses causes peripheral vasodilatation
  C   increases renal blood flow
  D   increases ventricular excitability
  E   increases splanchnic blood flow.

II.13   The following are true of α-adrenoceptor blocking agents:

  A   they increase blood flow in normal skin and muscle
  B   they cause drowsiness
  C   the clinically useful drugs are competitive antagonists
  D   they have only α_1-blocking activity
  E   they are chronotropic agents.

II.14 Diazepam:

A is an anticonvulsant
B acts on the limbic system
C can be metabolised to oxazepam
D has a half-life of less than 6 h
E can relax skeletal muscle.

II.15 The following are bronchodilators:

A salbutamol
B sodium cromoglycate
C isoflurane
D doxapram
E theophylline.

II.16 The following are properties of anaesthetic vapours:

A diethyl ether is a marked respiratory depressant during induction of anaesthesia
B halothane decreases cerebral blood flow
C isoflurane is soluble in rubber
D enflurane is a halogenated hydrocarbon
E nitrous oxide has a MAC of 101%.

II.17   **A base with a pK of 9:**

   A   will be strongly ionised in the stomach
   B   will be 75% ionised at a pH of 4.5
   C   is better excreted in an acid urine
   D   has maximum buffering power in a medium of pH 9
   E   has a titration curve described by the Bronsted–Lowry
       equation.

II.18   **Prochlorperazine:**

   A   is a phenothiazine
   B   can precipitate extrapyramidal reactions
   C   should not be given in pregnancy
   D   produces mild α-adrenergic blockade
   E   acts on the chemoreceptor trigger zone.

II.19   **Methods of prolonging the action of an equivalent dose of lignocaine include:**

   A   the addition of adrenaline
   B   carbonation
   C   using a more concentrated solution
   D   mixing with dextran in saline
   E   increasing the volume of drug injected.

II.20   **Cocaine:**

   A   competes with noradrenaline at binding sites
   B   causes vomiting
   C   depresses respiration
   D   hypersensitivity is rare
   E   is largely excreted unchanged in urine.

II.21   **The following interfere with blood grouping or incompatibility testing:**

   A   dextran 40
   B   warfarin
   C   dipyridamole
   D   aspirin
   E   tranexamic acid.

II.22   **In the cryoprobe:**

   A   cooling is an adiabatic process
   B   rapid gas expansion from a capillary tube produces a fall in temperature
   C   cooling is due to energy loss resulting from gas expansion
   D   carbon dioxide is a suitable gas for routine use
   E   tip temperatures as low as $-90°C$ are required for efficient use.

II.23 Which of the following statements about statistics are true:

A   the null hypothesis states that there is nothing to be gained
    from treatment
B   the significance level is a probability value that ensures the
    outcome is clinically significant
C   the standard deviation is a measure of the central tendency
    of the sample
D   the standard error allows a measured value to be related to
    its true value in the population
E   blood pressure is measured on an ordinal scale.

**II.24 The rise in alveolar concentration of anaesthetic agents is
more rapid:**

A   when the inspired concentration is higher
B   when the alveolar ventilation is increased
C   when the cardiac output is increased
D   when the agent is more soluble
E   when nitrous oxide is added to the inspired mixture.

**II.25 The following statements about osmotic phenomena are
true:**

A   the plasma osmotic pressure is 7 atmospheres
B   osmolality is stated as osmoles per kilogram of solvent
C   osmolality can be measured by depression of melting point
    of a liquid
D   the mathematical description of osmosis is analogous to the
    gas laws
E   osmosis occurs when two fluids are separated by a
    permeable membrane.

II.26 pH can be measured with:

A   a silver–silver chloride bridge electrode
B   a mercury half cell
C   a calomel half cell
D   a glass electrode
E   a platinum electrode.

II.27 Carbon dioxide in a mixture of gases may be measured by:
  A fuel cell
  B manometric van Slyke apparatus
  C Haldane apparatus
  D infra-red gas analyser
  E Severinghaus electrode.

II.28 The following statements about critical temperature are true:
  A it is the temperature above which a substance cannot be liquefied however much pressure is applied
  B the critical temperature of oxygen is $-119°C$
  C nitrous oxide cylinders will always contain liquid nitrous oxide
  D the critical temperature of nitrous oxide is $48.5°C$
  E at a substance's critical temperature, the vapour pressure is the critical pressure.

II.29 When a solid is mixed with a liquid:
  A compounds containing both highly hydrophobic and highly polar groups are termed antipathetic
  B only ionically charged compounds will dissolve in a polar medium such as water
  C heat may be absorbed from the surroundings
  D a colloid may be separated from a crystalloid by dialysis
  E solutions of similar molar concentration exert the same osmotic pressure.

II.30 For an exponential process:
  A the time constant is the natural logarithm of the half-life
  B the rate of the process is highest when the process begins
  C a plot on semi-logarithmic paper will give a straight line
  D an example would be unaided, passive exhalation
  E the time for a two-fold change in the current value is a constant.

Paper II Answers

II.1 **FTFTF**

A End-organ stimulation is adrenergic, but neurotransmission in the ganglion is cholinergic in both sympathetic and parasympathetic nervous systems.

C The grey rami communicantes link sympathetic ganglia to the spinal cord. The parasympathetic ganglia are supplied by cranial nerves III, VII, IX, X and XI, and sacral outflow.

E Lumbar sympathectomy is a method of pain relief.

II.2 **TFFFF**

B Although the heart valves are affected by contraction of ventricular muscle and the papillary muscles, the valves open and close because of the pressure gradients across them.

C Left ventricular pressure is approaching aortic *diastolic* pressure just before the aortic valve opens. Maximal pressure is systolic pressure.

D The ejection fraction is about 65%.

E The dicrotic notch is due to rebound of the elastic tissue of the *aorta*, not to rebound of the aortic valve.

II.3 **TTTFF**

A This is the origin of cor pulmonale in chronic bronchitics and right heart failure in 'blue babies'.

B Approximately the same flow passes through both circulations, but mean pulmonary pressure is about 15 mmHg while mean systemic arterial pressure is about 90 mmHg. By analogy with Ohm's law, resistance must be equivalently less.

C To measure resistance one must know the pressure differential and the flow; both can be measured with this catheter, though remember that not all pulmonary wedge catheters incorporate a thermistor.

D False: isoprenaline may reduce pulmonary artery pressure (decrease resistance) without affecting cardiac output.

E The effect of 5-HT on smooth muscle is complex. There is vasoconstriction or vasodilation depending on the particular vascular bed, the resting tone, and the dose of drug. There are also reflex effects, and effects on ganglionic transmission. The pulmonary vascular resistance increases sharply in dogs and cats, but less so in man.

D and **E** are pharmacology, in a physiology question. There may be questions such as these in the examination, especially in questions about the autonomic nervous system.

II.4   TFTTF

B   A cutaneous sensory receptor responds to a single
modality – because of **C**.
E   Stretch receptors are slowly-adapting.

II.5   TFTFT

B   There is negative feedback from the adrenal cortex.
D   Pancreatic secretions are controlled by locally released
hormones, for example secretin and pancreozymin.

II.6   FTTFT

A   The myenteric nerve plexus must be intact.
B   A wave of depolarisation passes through the longitudinal
muscle about 10 times per minute.
C   The myenteric reflex initiates a peristaltic wave.
D   VIP is a regulator of secretion. The use of the adjective
potent means that **D** will remain false even if someone
somewhere describes an effect of VIP on an isolated
segment of bowel in an experiment. Remember that this
examination is about a good understanding of basic
principles, not the minutiae of the latest research.
E   This causes the reflex ileus of peritoneal irritation.

II.7   FTFFT

A   Careful! Insulin is an *endocrine* secretion.
C,D   False. The main control is hormonal, but vagal stimulation
increases enzyme-rich secretion. This effect, but not the
effects of the hormones, is blocked by atropine.
E   Similarly to other systems in which precursors are
converted to active forms, for example the coagulation
cascade, inhibitors maintain a balance and prevent
runaway positive feedback.

II.8   FTTTF

A   ECF:ICF for sodium is 145:12.
B   ECF:ICF for magnesium is 2:15.
C   ECF:ICF for protein is 15:60.
D   ECF:ICF for pH is 7.4:7.0.
E   ECF:ICF for bicarbonate is 27.8.

II.9   **TFTFF**

B   Breathing 100% oxygen at sea-level depresses respiration initially, then there is a slight stimulation secondary to reflex changes in cerebral blood flow.

D   Oxygen equilibration will be complete unless exercise is severe, or there is anaemia, or there is a block to diffusion.

E   The gasping (at least in animals) is a chemoreceptor reflex.

II.10   **FFFTF**

A   False: though there may be these concentrations in the blood of heavy smokers.

B   Methaemoglobin forms in normal man but is reduced by the NADH–metHb reductase system.

C   Haemoglobin is not found free in the circulation.

E   False: 25% reduced Hb is equivalent to a PaO_2 of 40 mmHg – venous blood.

II.11   **FTTTT**

A   Hypercapnia and acidosis shift the curve to the right.

D   Decreases in 2,3-DPG shift the curve to the left; hypercapnia shifts it in the opposite direction.

II.12   **TFTTT**

A   Dopamine is inotropic and chronotropic.

B   In high doses it is an α-agonist.

C,E   There are specific dopaminergic receptors that subserve vasodilation in the kidney and mesentery.

II.13   **TTFFF**

A   The effect on blood flow in these organs depends on the prevailing sympathetic tone.

C   Phenoxybenzamine is not a competitive inhibitor.

D   Subdivision of α-receptors is not as clear, not are the clinical implications so obvious, as the subdivision of β-receptors. At the time of writing, this subject is being researched intensively because of the suggested link between α_2-receptors and anaesthesia.

E   They may cause reflex tachycardia.

II.14   TTTFT

B   The benzodiazepines affect the hippocampus, and other areas, quite selectively, on specific receptors.

C   This is small print. Diazepam *can* be metabolised to oxazepam but it is via an intermediate, it is species-specific and oxazepam has a shorter half-life than diazepam. It is of more importance to know when a metabolite has a longer half-life (for example, pentobarbitone from thiopentone).

D   The half-life of diazepam is 20–90 h (of oxazepam, incidentally, is 3–21 h).

E   Relaxation of skeletal muscle is not a direct action, but by actions at supraspinal loci.

II.15   TFTFT

A   Salbutamol is a β_2-stimulant.

B   Cromoglycate stabilises mast cell membranes and so reduces histamine release.

C   Isoflurane may cause irritation and an increase of secretions, but it is a smooth muscle relaxant.

D   Doxapram is effectively a centrally acting respiratory stimulant, though there is evidence that it acts on the peripheral arterial chemoreceptors.

II.16   FFTFF

Apparently straightforward questions may need to be treated with care.

A   Diethyl ether is a respiratory depressant at high concentrations, but a stimulant at lower concentrations.

B   Halothane causes cerebral vasodilation and increased flow.

C   Methoxyflurane is the agent most usually regarded as soluble in rubber, but other vapours have the same property.

D   Enflurane is a halogenated ether.

E   We do not wish to make candidates too paranoid, but it is important, particularly when considering topics in physics, to get your terminology correct. Nitrous oxide is a gas not a vapour (a vapour is defined as a gas below its critical temperature). The statement in branch **E** is true, but not when connected to the stem of the question. This is a bit harsh, but the idea of this book is to make you think a bit.

N_2O at rm temp would be a vapor

II.17   TFTTF

An important topic, about which questions can be confusing because of the wording. Try to think it through logically: pK is the pH at 50% ionisation, and acids tend to ionise in solutions of relative alkalinity (and vice versa).

E   Bronsted and Lowry defined an acid as a proton donor and a base as a proton acceptor; the shape of the titration curve is described by the Henderson–Hasselbalch equation.

II.18   TTFTT

A,B   All phenothiazines can precipitate extrapyramidal reactions.

C   Phenothiazine anti-emetics are not contraindicated in pregnancy.

II.19   TFTTT

B   False: adding sodium bicarbonate increases the rate of onset, but not the duration of action.

C,E   Both are true for epidural application, though probably not for local nerve blocks.

II.20   TTFFF

C   Cocaine is a respiratory stimulant, increasing rate rather than depth.

D   Hypersensitivity is common. Many people routinely test for hypersensitivity.

E   It is mainly metabolised, but a small amount is excreted unchanged.

II.21   TFFFF

A   All dextrans interfere with blood grouping or incompatibility testing, particularly those of high molecular weight.

B,C,D,E   All of these drugs affect coagulation, but not cross-matching.

E   Mefenamic acid (an aspirin-like drug) interferes. Methyl dopa and penicillin in high dose are two other common drugs that may interfere.

II.22   TTTTF

B   The principle of the cryoprobe is that gas expands rapidly after leaving a capillary tube and produces a decrease in temperature.

D   Although nitrous oxide is often used, carbon dioxide is equally suitable.

E   The lowest tip temperature achievable is − 70°C.

II.23   FFFTT

A   False. The null hypothesis is that the samples being tested are from the same population: it is a statistical, not a clinical, statement.

B   False. This is of prime importance. Statistical and clinical significance must not be confused.

C   The standard deviation is a measure of the variability.

D   Confidence intervals (around the measured value) are calculated from the standard error.

II.24   TTFFT

C   The alveolar concentration increases more quickly when cardiac output is reduced, increased output removing gas more quickly.

D   A soluble drug passes into blood more readily, which reduces the alveolar concentration. Thus the alveolar partial pressure takes longer to rise.

E   This is the second gas effect, whereby rapid uptake of nitrous oxide increases the alveolar concentration of other gases present.

II.25   TTTTF

A   This is the *total* osmotic pressure; oncotic pressure is the effective osmotic pressure and is much less (25 mmHg).

B   Osmolality is defined as osmoles per kilogram of solvent, while osmolarity is per litre of solution.

D   The ideal gas equation ($PV = nRT$) applies.

E   Osmosis occurs when the membrane is *semi*permeable preventing some molecules equilibrating down their concentration gradients.

II.26   FFFTF

The mercury and calomel half-cells are constituents of electrode systems; silver–silver chloride and platinum electrodes are used for recording various biological potentials. Only the glass electrode can measure pH.

II.27   FFTTT

A   False: fuel cells measure oxygen.

B   The van Slyke apparatus is a difficult, time-consuming method of measuring the volumes of carbon dioxide and oxygen in a sample of blood. It is inaccurate in the presence of anaesthetic gases.

C   A modification of the Haldane apparatus is still the absolute standard by which more sophisticated equipment is calibrated.

D   The infra-red gas analyser is now the clinical standard.

E   The Severinghaus electrode is a pH-sensitive electrode arranged to measure the pH of a thin film of bicarbonate covered by a gas-permeable Teflon membrane.

II.28   TTFFT

C   A nitrous oxide cylinder contains liquid nitrous oxide until all the liquid has vaporised (at about one-fifth full in normal, British, temperatures).

D   The critical temperature of nitrous oxide is 36.5°C.

II.29   FFTTF

A   These detergent-like molecules are said to be amphipathic.

B   Non-ionic compounds *dissolve;* polar – charged – compounds such as sugars and alcohols dissolve by forming hydrogen bonds with water.

C   When heat is absorbed during a chemical reaction, or during the dissolving of a solid in a liquid, it is termed endothermic.

D   A colloid consists of minute suspended particles mixed in a dispersion medium. A solution contains no particles.

E   The osmotic effect is a function of the number of particles in a solution. Thus dissociated sodium chloride exerts a greater osmotic pressure than an equimolar solution of a non-dissociated compound.

II.30   FTTTT

Time constant and half-life are two ways of describing the rate of an exponential process. The half-life is easier to understand and is stated in E. The time constant is about one and a half times the half-life and is best understood from a consideration of the mathematics of the exponential process; it is also the time in which the process would be completed if it were to continue at its initial rate.

time constant
≃ 1½ × t½ → time
Process would be
complete if it were
to continue at initial rate

t½ = time for 2 fold
change in current value
= constant.

other purines

↓

Hypoxanthine

xanthine
oxidase → uric acid

excreted in humans
in urine

98% filtered uric acid reabsorbed
tubular secretion

Urea cycle

Aspartate → Argininosuccinate → fumarate

Citrulline   Arginine

Pi

Casamoyl
phosphate   urea

Ornithine

$NH_4^+ \rightleftharpoons NH_3$

methionine
glycine   [liver]
arginine   ATP   skeletal muscle

creatine   rest   Phosphoryl creatine (energy store for
                                          ATP
                  creatine+ADP   synthesis)

            exercise
            reversed
            maintains
            supply of ATP
            immed source   creatinine
            of energy for
            muscle

Paper III Questions

III.1 **Compensatory mechanisms for a primary acidosis include:**
 A hyperventilation
 B increased urine pH
 C elevated cerebrospinal fluid bicarbonate
 D decreased carbonic anhydrase activity within the renal tubular cells
 E bicarbonate excretion to control urinary pH.

III.2 **In protein metabolism:**
 A methionine is a common source of methyl groups for synthesis
 B the urea cycle involves ornithine, citrulline and arginine
 C the urea cycle produces uric acid
 D creatinine is synthesised directly from creatine
 E essential amino acids are L-forms, non-essential are D-forms.

III.3 **In the normal cardiac cycle:**
 A the period of ventricular systole is equal to the Q–T interval
 B the duration of the QRS complex depends on the heart rate
 C the PR interval is less than 0.22 s
 D ejection occurs throughout systole
 E the R–R interval may vary.

III.4 **In the regulation of plasma potassium:**
 A potassium is actively secreted into tubular fluid
 B plasma concentrations are elevated acutely by an α-adrenergic effect
 C hyperkalaemia increases insulin secretion
 D mineralocorticoids cause hyperkalaemia
 E intracellular alkalosis decreases plasma potassium.

III.5 **The following are true of antidiuretic hormone:**
 A it is produced in the posterior lobe of the pituitary gland
 B its release is stimulated by a rise in plasma osmolarity
 C its release is stimulated by an increase in effective extracellular fluid volume
 D inappropriate release may occur during surgery
 E it is a vasoconstrictor in physiological concentrations.

III.6 **Dietary deficiencies of the following cause specific faults in erythropoiesis:**
A   ascorbic acid
B   folic acid
C   vitamin E
D   cyanocobalamin
E   valine.

III.7 **Cerebrospinal fluid:**
A   has a lower glucose content than blood
B   has a better buffering capacity than blood
C   has a normal cell count of 50–100 per cubic millimetre
D   is a clear yellow liquid
E   has a lower pH than plasma.

III.8 **Renin:**
A   is secreted from the juxta-glomerular cells
B   is released in response to a decrease in mean renal arterial blood pressure
C   is released in response to changes in sodium delivery to the kidney
D   has a half-life in the plasma of about an hour
E   acts on a precursor to form aldosterone.

III.9 **The oxygen carrying capacity of the blood is:**
A   the maximum quantity of oxygen that will combine with 100 ml of whole blood
B   the ratio between oxygen uptake and oxygen usage
C   independent of the haemoglobin concentration
D   the oxygen physically dissolved in blood
E   normally of the order of 15 ml per 100 ml whole blood.

III.10 **The following statements are true of the oxyhaemoglobin dissociation curve:**
A   the P_{50} is approximately 3.6 kPa (27 mmHg)
B   the curve moves to the left if there is hypocapnia
C   the curve moves to the right if there is alkalosis
D   the P_{50} is decreased by a raised $PaCO_2$
E   the steepest part of the curve is below the normal venous point.

III.11 **There are separate sensory receptors for:**
A   pain
B   light touch
C   two-point discrimination
D   vibration
E   cold.

III.12   Atrial natriuretic peptide:

- **A**   has not yet been isolated but its assumed existence explains certain physiological phenomena
- **B**   causes relaxation of mesangial glomerular cells
- **C**   is a physiological antagonist to angiotensin II
- **D**   secretion is increased when dietary sodium is increased
- **E**   is released when atrial muscle is stretched.

III.13   Phosphodiesterase inhibitors:

- **A**   increase the concentration of intracellular cyclic AMP
- **B**   are agonists at the β_1-adrenoceptor
- **C**   are positive inotropes
- **D**   depend on circulating catecholamines for their action
- **E**   include amiodarone.

III.14   Captopril:

- **A**   increases the rate of breakdown of angiotensin II
- **B**   inhibits the breakdown of bradykinin
- **C**   may cause an increase in plasma potassium
- **D**   can safely be given in large doses in hypertensive crisis
- **E**   urine should be checked regularly for proteinuria.

III.15   The following drugs stimulate vasopressin secretion:

- **A**   morphine
- **B**   carbamazepine
- **C**   alcohol
- **D**   chlorpropamide
- **E**   dipyridamole.

III.16   Halothane:

- **A**   has a boiling point of 82°C
- **B**   has a saturated vapour pressure at 20°C of 343 mmHg
- **C**   is more soluble in blood than is isoflurane
- **D**   has trifluoroacetic acid as its major metabolite
- **E**   is stable on exposure to light.

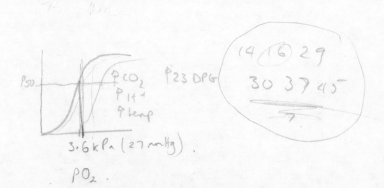

III.17 The following are isotonic with plasma:

A   1.2% sodium bicarbonate
B   5% dextrose
C   0.9 molar NaCl
D   Hartmann's solution (Ringer–Lactate)
E   human plasma protein fraction (5% human albumin solution).

III.18 Monoamine oxidase:

A   does not break down histamine
B   is inhibited by ephedrine
C   is synthesised in the placenta
D   occurs in highest concentrations in the body in the brain
E   metabolises noradrenaline that has leaked from storage
       granules.

III.19 Tubocurarine:

A   has ganglion-blocking effects
B   is antagonised by magnesium ions
C   does not cause histamine release
D   is partially inactivated before excretion
E   crosses the placenta in clinically important amounts.

III.20 Alfentanil:

A   is more potent than fentanyl
B   is largely non-ionised at plasma pH
C   is rapidly redistributed
D   has a small volume of distribution
E   causes chest wall rigidity.

III.21 Aminoglycoside antibiotics:

A   cannot be given orally
B   are inactive against *Staph. aureus*
C   are useful in severe infections presumed to be due to
       Pseudomonas aeruginosa
D   should be avoided in pregnancy
E   excretion is 50% renal.

III.22   Atropine:

- A   is cycloplegic
- B   decreases physiological dead space
- C   may induce hyperpyrexia in children
- D   may increase the incidence of halothane-induced dysrhythmias
- E   increases the likelihood of regurgitation on induction of anaesthesia.

III.23   Methoxamine:

- A   is a pure α-agonist
- B   has both direct and indirect effects at adrenergic receptors
- C   increases the irritability of heart muscle
- D   decreases cardiac output
- E   can only be given intravenously.

III.24   The following are true of these biological potentials:

- A   the normal signal amplitude of the electrocardiogram is of the order of 1 mV
- B   the frequency components of the ECG signal are between 0.5 and 80 Hz
- C   the normal signal amplitude of the EEG is of the order of microvolts
- D   electrical activity from muscle does not interfere with the electrocardiogram
- E   the electroencephalogram does not interfere with the ECG.

III.25   The closing volume:

- A   decreases with age
- B   is part of the functional residual capacity
- C   is greater when supine than when upright
- D   is measured by slow expiration of a marker gas
- E   is indicated on the tracer-volume curve at the transition between phases III and IV.

III.26   The Henderson–Hasselbalch equation:

- A   implies a constant ratio between carbon dioxide and bicarbonate
- B   includes a term for saturation of haemoglobin
- C   uses a pK of approximately 6.1
- D   applies only in vitro
- E   includes a term for buffer base.

III.27   The following are true of osmosis:

A   it is the basis of the red cell fragility test
B   the osmolarity of body fluids is mainly due to proteins
C   large molecules are more efficient generators of osmotic pressure
D   oncotic pressure is the effective osmotic pressure of the plasma
E   the pressure can be calculated by using Raoult's law.

III.28   When measuring arterial blood pressure using a sphygmomanometer cuff:

A   if the cuff is too small for the arm the pressure will tend to read high
B   accuracy is increased by leaving the cuff slightly inflated between readings
C   the slower the deflation, the more accurate the reading
D   a mercury column has a low frequency response
E   diastolic pressure agrees more accurately with direct measurement than will systolic pressure.

III.29   During intermittent positive pressure ventilation using a ventilator that is a constant flow generator:

A   the driving pressure is the difference between airway pressure and intrapleural pressure
B   the tidal volume is unaltered by changes in airways resistance
C   the tidal volume will depend on the compliance
D   alveolar pressure rises linearly during inspiration
E   peak airway pressure is reduced by having an inspiratory plateau, or 'hold'.

III.30   **In the international standard system of measurement (SI system):**

  A   the unit of time is the minute
  B   the unit of length is defined by a standard metre of iridium steel at constant temperature
  C   the unit of temperature is approximately the same magnitude as the centigrade degree
  D   the newton is the derived unit of force
  E   the bel is a unit of energy.

Paper III   Answers

III.1   **TTFFF**

A   The question does not qualify the acidosis. Remember that a primary respiratory acidosis is caused by hypoventilation.

C   Reduced bicarbonate increases respiratory drive.

D   Carbonic anhydrase activity increases; production and excretion of hydrogen ion is increased.

E   Hydrogen ions are excreted and the urine is acid.

III.2   **TTFFF**

C   Uric acid is a product of purine catabolism.

D   Creatinine is synthesised from phosphocreatine.

E   All amino acids found in nature are L-forms.

III.3   **TFTFT**

B,E   The Q–T interval depends on the heart rate; the R–R interval is the reciprocal of the rate; the QRS is unaffected by the rate.

D   There is no ejection during the phase of isovolumetric contraction.

III.4   **TTFTF**

A   Potassium is secreted into the fluid in the distal convoluted tubule, normally in amounts that balance intake.

D   Mineralocorticoids cause exchange of sodium for potassium (and hydrogen ions) in the renal tubules; potassium is lost.

E   True: potassium passes into cells and maintains electrical neutrality.

III.5   **TTFTF**

C   Release of antidiuretic hormone is stimulated by a decreased extracellular fluid volume.

E   Antidiuretic hormone is a vasoconstrictor in pharmacological concentrations.

III.6   FTFTF

Good nutrition is important for normal erythropoiesis and so a grossly deficient diet may affect red cell production in many ways. Cyanocobalamin (B_{12}) and folate both have an essential, specific place, unlike vitamin C. Vitamin E may be important in premature infants but certainly not in adults. Valine is an essential amino acid but that does not make it any more specifically involved with erythropoiesis than other essential amino acids — its replacement by glutamic acid in haemoglobin in sickle-cell anaemia is of genetic origin and is not caused by the non-availability of valine.

III.7   TFFFT

B,E   Lack of proteins means that buffering is less; hence the pH is lower.

C   There are up to three lymphocytes per cubic millimetre.

D   It is a clear, colourless liquid.

III.8   TTTTF

E   Renin acts on a circulating globulin to form angiotensin I.

III.9   TFFFF

C,D   The oxygen capacity depends largely upon oxygen combined with haemoglobin.

E   Assuming a haemoglobin concentration of 15 g/dl, the normal figure for oxygen carrying capacity is 20 ml/100 ml.

III.10   TTFFT

You must know the oxyhaemoglobin dissociation curve. In an MCQ exam it is helpful to draw the curve on scrap paper before answering the question: the wording can be very confusing because the same condition can be presented in so many ways — for instance, (B) and (D) are both the effect of carbon dioxide.

III.11   TTFFT

C,D   Two-point discrimination and vibration sense are composite sensations for which the initial stimulus is signalled by touch receptors.

III.12   FTTTT

A   Atrial natriuretic peptide was for many years a theoretical explanation for physiological observations. The peptide has now been characterised for a number of species.

III.13   TFTFF

B,C,D   Phosphodiesterase inhibitors bypass circulating catecholamines and β_1-receptors

E   Amiodarone is an anti-arrhythmic drug; amrinone is the phosphodiesterase inhibitor.

III.14   FTTFT

A   Captopril inhibits the enzyme that converts angiotensin I to angiotensin II.

D   Initial treatment must be with care, to avoid severe hypotension.

E   Proteinuria occurs in about 1 in 200 patients, more if there is pre-existing renal disease.

III.15   TTFTF

Pharmacological agents that stimulate the secretion of ADH are believed to be cholinergic agonists, PGE_1 (although this inhibits its action on the kidney), and large doses of barbiturates. Morphine probably raises the threshold for secretion rather than actual release. β-agonists cause antidiuresis; α-agonists cause diuresis.

   One cannot know every effect of every drug. You may be lucky and pick up a mark for an occasional remembered connection but don't guess if you don't know. You should have known morphine and alcohol (which decreases secretion).

E   Dipyridamole probably has no effect either way.

III.16   FFTTF

A,B   Halothane boils at 50°C and its saturated vapour pressure is 243 mmHg. Although halothane is less used now than formerly, as the first of the modern inhalational agents you must know about it.

E   Halothane is stabilised with thymol.

III.17 TFFTT

A   The more usual 8.4% sodium bicarbonate is strongly hypertonic.

B   5% dextrose is *isosmolar*, but uptake of the sugar by the red cells soon renders 5% dextrose effectively hypotonic and the red cells lyse.

C   0.9M (molar) NaCl would be extremely hypertonic. A molar solution of NaCl contains 58.5 grams per litre. Remember that chemical and physiological 'normality' are not the same. 0.9% NaCl is isotonic (9 g/l).

III.18 TTTFT

A   Histamine itself is broken down by di-amine oxidase (histaminase) and the resulting methyl-histamine is metabolised by monoamine oxidase.

D   The highest concentrations of monoamine oxidase are in the liver.

III.19 TFFTF

B   Tubocurarine is antagonised in vitro by Ca^{2+}; and Ca^{2+} and Mg^{2+} usually have opposing actions.

D   One-third in urine, some in bile, some metabolised.

III.20 FTTTT

A   Potency is a description of effect per dose. It is independent of rapidity of onset or duration of action. For an equivalent effect, you need ten times as much alfentanil.

B   Whatever arguments are used about semi-quantitative words like 'largely', alfentanil is only about 10% ionised. (It is a base with a low pKa, and is therefore a weak base that 'sees' the plasma as alkali and can only reluctantly accept protons.)

D   Although cleared more slowly than fentanyl by the liver, the small volume of distribution means that it is eliminated more quickly.

III.21 FFTTF

A   Aminoglycosides are not absorbed from the gastrointestinal tract so there is no point in giving them orally for *systemic* infection. They *can* be given orally to control intestinal bacteria.

D   They should not be given in pregnancy because of fetal ototoxicity.

E   Excretion is entirely renal.

III.22   TFTTT

A   Cycloplegia is paralysis of accommodation.
B   Atropine decreases saturation by increasing physiological dead space.
E   It reduces the integrity of the cardiac sphincter. This is one of the mechanisms by which atropine makes metoclopramide a less effective anti-emetic.

III.23   TTFTF

C   Cardiac irritability is not increased and methoxamine can safely be used during anaesthesia with volatile agents.
E   Methoxamine can be given intramuscularly for a more sustained effect.

III.24   TTTFT

B   The frequency components of a signal are important when designing suitable amplifiers, to avoid distortion of the signal. Similar considerations are important to anaesthetists when looking at the shape of the arterial blood pressure waveform.
D,E The disturbance caused by shivering or other tremors is partly movement but partly direct electrical interference. Electroencephalographic signals are of too low voltage to interfere with the electrocardiogram.

III.25   FFTTT

A   The closing volume *increases* with age.
B   The closing volume is independent of the functional residual capacity. It may be larger or smaller.
E   You should be able to draw, and to understand, the plot of tracer concentration against volume obtained from this test.

III.26   FFTFF

If you can *derive* the Henderson–Hasselbalch equation you will understand it better than if you only learn it.

A   The implication is that the pH *depends* on the ratio, not that it is constant.

III.27   TFFTF

A   The normal red cell will lyse in saline more dilute than about 0.4–0.45%.

B   The osmolarity of body fluids is due mainly to ions.

C   This is a trap: large molecules cannot pass out of the circulating volume so easily and so are more effective at retaining fluid within it, but osmotic pressure is generated by the number of particles, unrelated to their size.

D   Oncotic pressure is due to proteins.

E   Raoult's law: the depression of vapour pressure of a solvent is proportional to the molar concentration of the solute.

III.28   TFTTF

A   The pressure will not be transmitted fully to the artery: as a rough guide the cuff should cover one-third to one-half of the upper arm from elbow to shoulder.

B   Venous engorgement reduces accuracy.

C   Only up to a point because the stimulus of the inflated cuff will raise the blood pressure and increase venous engorgement.

E   Systolic pressure agrees better. Agreement with diastolic pressure is complicated by differences in which of the Korotkoff sounds is deemed to correspond to the diastolic pressure.

III.29   FTFTF

A,B,C The driving pressure of a constant flow generator is generally set by the pressure relief valve of the ventilator, and will only reach this pressure if the resistance is excessively high or the compliance excessively low. Unless that happens, tidal volume is unaffected.

E   Peak pressure occurs at the end of the active phase of inspiration; an inspiratory plateau can have no direct effect. If there is an inspiratory hold at a given I:E ratio, the peak pressure will actually be higher, unless the set tidal volume is reduced.

III.30 **FFTTF**

A   The SI unit of time is the second.

B   The SI unit of length is the metre, but is defined using the wavelength of a particular emission of electromagnetic radiation (krypton-86).

C   The unit of temperature is the kelvin, and 1°K is virtually the same as 1°C.

D   The unit of force (N: the newton) is mass × acceleration = $kg.m.s^{-2}$. The SI unit of pressure is the pascal, which is $N.m^{-2}$.

E   The bel is a unit for describing power ratios. It is a logarithmic description, so a ratio of 10:1 is 1 bel, and 3 dB is a ratio of 2:1.

Paper IV Questions

IV.1 Sympathetic innervation of blood vessels:
- **A** is mediated by α-adrenoceptors
- **B** is mediated locally by noradrenaline
- **C** implies that sympathectomy induces vasodilation
- **D** increases flow independent of vessel diameter
- **E** induces vasodilation in response to cold and haemorrhage.

IV.2 Venous return to the heart is decreased by:
- **A** the Valsalva manoeuvre
- **B** exercise
- **C** paralysis of skeletal muscles
- **D** femoral arterio–venous fistula
- **E** rapid infusion of blood.

IV.3 The following are true of nerve conduction:
- **A** the amplitude of the action potential is determined by the equilibrium potential for sodium
- **B** the duration of the absolute refractory period is of the order of a millisecond
- **C** the length of the refractory period limits transmission frequency
- **D** conduction is faster in myelinated fibres
- **E** saltatory conduction involves sodium and chloride permeability alone.

IV.4 Insulin has the following actions in skeletal muscle:
- **A** enhancement of glycogen synthesis
- **B** enhancement of uptake of amino acids
- **C** increase in protein synthesis
- **D** increase in production of ketones
- **E** increase in phosphorylation of glucose.

IV.5 Serum albumin:
- **A** is synthesised mainly in the reticuloendothelial system
- **B** has a half-life in the circulation of approximately 3 days
- **C** is generally normal in acute liver disease
- **D** is 5–10% higher in the recumbent than in the upright position
- **E** is increased 10–20% after prolonged venous stasis.

IV.6 **The following are important in physiological limitation of blood clotting:**
A   removal of activated clotting factors by the liver
B   prostacyclin
C   protein C
D   a factor released from the endothelial cells
E   fibrinogen.

IV.7 **In the nephron:**
A   all membranes are equally permeable to water
B   two-thirds of the glomerular filtrate is absorbed in the proximal convoluted tubule
C   the medulla has an osmolarity of 1200 mosmol/l
D   sodium is exchanged for potassium in the distal convoluted tubule
E   the collecting ducts form a countercurrent multiplier.

IV.8 **At high altitude, pulmonary ventilation increases because of:**
A   the direct effect of lower barometric pressure
B   decreased alveolar carbon dioxide tension
C   decreased compliance
D   increased oxygen consumption
E   the development of pulmonary oedema.

IV.9 **In acute tissue hypoxia:**
A   dyspnoea combined with hyperpnoea is diagnostic
B   there is tachycardia
C   the blood pressure is likely to be increased
D   respiratory stimulation is from the peripheral chemoreceptors
E   there will be cyanosis.

IV.10 **At functional residual capacity:**
A   a healthy subject should be able to breath-hold for at least 25 s
B   the tendency of the chest wall to expand is exactly balanced by the tendency of the lungs to collapse
C   ventilation–perfusion ratios are optimal
D   static compliance is minimal
E   the lungs still contain the expiratory reserve volume and the residual volume.

IV.11 Deoxyribosenucleic acid:

    A replicates in the cell nucleus by the polymerase chain reaction
    B acts as template for the formation of messenger RNA
    C is formed by the aggregation of transfer RNA
    D is directly responsible for protein synthesis
    E is a double helix.

IV.12 The following are true of antacids:

    A magnesium trisilicate is soluble in gastric acid
    B aluminium hydroxide acts rapidly
    C sodium citrate causes transient metabolic alkalosis
    D aluminium hydroxide is contraindicated in renal failure
    E they tend to stimulate acid secretion.

IV.13 The following are anticonvulsants:

    A midazolam
    B suxamethonium
    C chlormethiazole
    D thiopentone
    E trifluoperazine.

IV.14 Sodium nitroprusside:

    A acts as a postsynaptic inhibitory transmitter
    B causes dilated pupils
    C is broken down to nitric oxide in the plasma
    D when given as a prolonged infusion may cause persistent lactic acidosis
    E should not be given with β-blockers.

IV.15 Methohexitone:

    A is more potent than thiopentone
    B can cause pain on injection
    C can cause excitatory movements
    D is an anticonvulsant
    E is unstable in solution.

IV.16 A drug that is strongly protein-bound:

    A will be metabolised rapidly
    B may interfere with the pharmacodynamics of warfarin
    C will induce liver microsomal enzymes
    D will cause an increase in the serum albumin
    E will have a relatively low 'free' concentration in the plasma.

IV.17 Which of the following are true:

A   alkalinisation of the urine increases the excretion of phenobarbitone

B   acidification of the urine reduces aspirin elimination

C   hydrogen ion excretion in the kidney is dependent upon carbonic anhydrase activity

D   acetazolamide therapy may produce hypokalaemia

E   elective hyperventilation increases hydrogen ion excretion.

IV.18 Central effects of lignocaine include:

A   sedation

B   convulsions

C   vomiting

D   tachycardia

E   tinnitus.

IV.19 The following are true of acetylcholinesterase:

A   it is present in red blood cells

B   the anionic site binds the N^+ atom of acetylcholine

C   the enzyme is acetylated when acetylcholine is hydrolysed

D   it is inhibited by neostigmine

E   physiological acetylation of the enzyme is a short-lived phenomenon.

IV.20 The following have interactions likely to be of clinical importance:

A   propranolol and ergotamine

B   metformin and alcohol

C   pancuronium and carbenicillin

D   diclofenac and angiotensin converting enzyme inhibitors

E   oral iron and chloramphenicol.

IV.21 Heart rate is slowed by:

A   amphetamine

B   atropine

C   propranolol

D   dobutamine

E   nifedipine.

IV.22   Using propranolol to treat hypertension:

   A may exacerbate asthma
   B often produces postural hypotension
   C is contraindicated in patients with high plasma renin levels
   D may precipitate cardiac failure in susceptible patients
   E should be avoided in a patient with Raynaud's phenomenon.

IV.23   Cardiac output may be measured by:

   A thermodilution
   B electromagnetic flow meter
   C Doppler ultrasound
   D limb plethysmography
   E ballistocardiography.

IV.24   In pulse oximetry:

   A the theoretical basis is Stefan's law
   B calibration is against known in vitro standards
   C carboxyhaemoglobin does not affect readings
   D accuracy at readings above 90% saturation is to within 0.1%
   E pulse amplitude is a good indicator of cardiac output.

IV.25   The following statements about statistics are true:

   A the unpaired t-test is a test of the difference between sample means
   B the standard deviation decreases with the size of sample
   C the Chi-squared test applies to nominal data
   D the Normal (Gaussian) distribution is asymmetrical
   E correlation indicates causation.

IV.26 In the measurement of renal function:
- A   inulin is used because it is completely cleared by the glomeruli
- B   creatinine clearance is approximately the same as inulin clearance
- C   glomerular filtration is inversely proportional to the blood urea
- D   up to 750 mg of protein may be lost daily through normal kidneys
- E   the normal serum creatinine is less than 133 µmol/l.

IV.27 In a consideration of whether flow is laminar or turbulent:
- A   Reynolds number is an index of the type of flow
- B   critical velocity is a constant for a particular fluid
- C   helium is less dense than nitrogen
- D   laminar flow is more likely with a more viscous fluid
- E   turbulent flow within blood vessels causes a bruit.

IV.28 In a nerve stimulator used to locate nerves or to monitor train-of-four:
- A   current passed is between 10 and 100 milliamps
- B   the tetanic frequency is usually 50 or 100 Hz
- C   electrode jelly is used to reduce skin resistance
- D   higher current is necessary with subcutaneous needle electrodes
- E   the electrical impulse is a square wave.

IV.29 The amount of a gas that dissolves in a liquid in physical solution:
- A   will increase if the temperature decreases
- B   is defined by the partition coefficient
- C   is inversely proportional to the partial pressure
- D   is governed by Henry's law
- E   can be calculated from the Fick principle.

IV.30 **The following are true of heat and temperature:**
  A temperature is a form of energy
  B resistance wire can be used for small temperature changes
  C thermistors have a fast response time
  D thermocouples depend on the Seebeck effect
  E the triple point of water is used to construct the kelvin scale.

$$R_e = \frac{D\,R}{V}$$

Paper IV   Answers

IV.1   TTTFF

D   Flow is dependent on vessel diameter if the pressure differential remains constant.

E   Cold and haemorrhage induce vasoconstriction.

IV.2   TFTFF

A   Venous return decreases at the onset of the manoeuvre.

B   Exercise increases cardiac output.

C   Loss of the 'muscle pump' reduces venous return.

D   Cardiac output will increase to compensate for the shunt.

E   Rapid infusion simulates venous return.

IV.3   TTTTF

B   The absolute refractory period is 0.4–1.0 ms.

C   In sympathetic fibres the refractory period is 2 ms.

E   Saltatory conduction refers to transmission that proceeds via the nodes of Ranvier, not to salt!

IV.4   TTTFF

Insulin is the main hormone of anabolism. It is extremely important and you should be clear about its many actions. Flow charts and diagrams are helpful.

D   It enhances *uptake* of ketones.

E   Phosphorylation of glucose is controlled by other hormones. The rapid phosphorylation maintains the concentration gradient for glucose across the cell membrane.

IV.5   TFFFF

B   The half-life of albumin in the circulation is 17–26 d.

D   Don't get muddled up with orthostatic proteinuria.

E   The question doesn't state whether the increase of serum albumin is systemic, or a local effect distal to the site of occlusion. The answer is 'false' anyway.

IV.6   TTTTF

B   Prostacyclin is the physiological antagonist of thromboxane A_2 on platelet function.

C   Thrombin activates protein C (indirectly). Congenital absence of protein C is usually fatal.

D   This factor is thrombomodulin, the factor that converts thrombin into protein C activator.

E   Fibrinogen is not directly involved in fibrinolysis.

IV.7   FTTTF

It is beyond the scope of this book fully to explain the workings of the nephron – but it is very important. The counter-current system in particular needs clear thinking: the loops of Henle are described as countercurrent multipliers, the vasa recta as countercurrent exchangers.

IV.8   FFFFF

A   Ventilation increases because of the indirect effect that barometric pressure decreases and reduces inspired oxygen.

B PCO_2 is decreased because of hyperventilation.

C,E   Pulmonary oedema is not part of the physiological response to high altitude. If oedema develops, compliance decreases; but that here is a red herring.

IV.9   FTFTF

A   'Diagnostic' means that these symptoms could only be of hypoxia, and that is obviously untrue.

B   An early sign and more reliable than hypertension.

C,D   Stimulation of the peripheral chemoreceptors causes increased ventilation. Reflex hypertension is likely but not inevitable. Eventually, if severe or protracted enough, there will be circulatory collapse.

E   Not always: not, for instance, in severe anaemia, carbon monoxide poisoning or cyanide poisoning.

IV.10   TTFFT

C   In elderly, though normal, subjects, some airways will be closed at FRC. Even in younger patients it is unlikely to be true: if 'optimal' means unity then it is never true; if it means the best possible then it will remain so for a good range of lung expansion above FRC.

D   Compliance is least at total lung capacity. It is greatest over a range of 1–2 litres above FRC.

Thermodynamic Theory (handwritten note)

IV.11   FTFFT

Protein C → activated protein (handwritten note)

A   The polymerase chain reaction is a biochemical
      technique by which multiple copies of DNA are
      obtained.

B,C,D The process of m-RNA formation is *transcription*.
      Transfer RNA carries amino acids to the m-RNA. Protein
      synthesis is thus a few steps removed from DNA.

E   DNA is *the* double helix. You might ask why
      anaesthetists should know about these aspects of
      physiology, which seem remote from clinical practice.
      The 'new genetics' are likely to affect every specialty.

IV.12   FFTTT

A,C   Magnesium trisilicate (and aluminium hydroxide) are
      favoured because they are insoluble and less likely to
      cause systemic acid-base disturbances.

B   Most insoluble antacids act slowly (sometimes more
      slowly than gastric emptying!).

D   Aluminium is excreted in the urine.

IV.13   TFTTF

B   Suxamethonium prevents the muscular manifestations
      only.

E   Trifluoperazine is a piperazine phenothiazine used as a
      long-acting major tranquilliser.

IV.14   FFTTF

(C) → False · SNP/GTN converted to NO in vasc sm muscle cell (handwritten note)

A   Sodium nitroprusside acts directly on smooth muscle.

B   Ganglion blockers, no longer as popular as they once
      were for hypotensive anaesthesia, dilate the pupils.

E   Beta-blockers may have to be given, especially to the
      young, to prevent troublesome reflex tachycardia. *(Calvey Williams)* (handwritten note)

IV.15   TTTFF

A   Potency is a misused word that means, strictly, the
      weight-for-weight effectiveness of a drug and says
      nothing about speed of action.

C,D   Muscular movements on induction are not necessarily
      epileptiform, but methohexitone does have convulsant
      activity in those prone to epilepsy.

IV.16   FTFFT

A   Only free drug can be metabolised.

B   The drug will displace warfarin and increase the effect of
      a given dose.

C,D   There is no connection.

Pharmacokinetics. (handwritten note)

IV.17 TTTTF

A   True: phenobarbitone is more ionised in alkaline urine, which reduces its reabsorption.

B   True: the opposite of **A**.

D   Potassium ions are excreted in preference to hydrogen ions.

E   Renal compensation for respiratory alkalosis decreases hydrogen ion excretion.

IV.18 TTFFT

C   Not a feature of lignocaine overdose.

D   There is bradycardia.

IV.19 TTTTT

D   This must be one of the easiest questions in the book.

E   The acetylated enzyme is stable for a few microseconds. The enzyme is reformed by hydrolysis, with the release of acetic acid.

IV.20 TTFTF

A   Propranolol and ergotamine both cause peripheral vasoconstriction.

B   The risk with metformin and alcohol is lactic acidosis.

C   The interaction at the neuromuscular junction is with the aminoglycosides and some of the less commonly used antibiotics.

D   The combination can produce renal impairment.

E   Iron chelates tetracyclines, not chloramphenicol.

IV.21 FFTFF

A   Amphetamine in normal dosage does not usually affect heart rate, but slight tachycardia is possible.

B   Vagal blockade by atropine produces tachycardia. Atropine can produce a centrally mediated bradycardia, but it is rarely marked.

D   Dobutamine is said to increase cardiac output without affecting rate.

E   The acute response to nifedipine is an increase in rate, which then settles back to normal.

IV.22   TFFTT

A   Propranolol is non-selective: bronchial relaxation is β_2.
B   The vasodilatory antihypertensives are likely to cause postural hypotension.
C   Propranolol is particularly useful with high renin levels and actually decreases its production, though the ACE-inhibitors are now more likely to be prescribed.
E   Propranolol can inhibit peripheral vasodilatation.

IV.23   TTTFT

A   Thermodilution is now used routinely in many intensive care units.
B   Electromagnetic flow meters are much used in research, especially animal research.
D   Limb plethysmography measures blood flow to the limb.
E   Ballistocardiography is now outmoded, but its physical principles are important.

IV.24   FFFFF

Pulse oximetry is now a standard, almost essential, monitor and you must know its limitations. We can allow that you might not have known that the theoretical basis of absorption of light is the Lambert–Beer Law. (Stefan's law describes radiation from black bodies.) But there is little excuse for getting any other branch of this question wrong.

B   One of the problems of pulse oximetry is a lack of a reliable in vitro calibration.
C   High concentrations of carboxyhaemoglobin cause pulse oximeters to over-read.
D   Accuracy is to 2% at best.
E   Pulse amplitude is *an* indicator, but cannot be described as a *good* indicator.

IV.25   TFTFF

B   The standard deviation increases with size of sample, though not much once the sample is greater than 10. The standard error of the mean decreases with size of sample.
D   The normal distribution is symmetrical.
E   Correlation indicates association, but not necessarily causation.

IV.26   FTFFT

A   Inulin is freely filtered at the glomeruli (which is not the same as completely cleared). It is a useful biochemical tool because it is neither secreted nor absorbed by the tubules.

C   Blood urea is unaffected until glomerular filtration is considerably reduced.

D   Up to 150 mg (not 750 mg) of protein may be lost daily.

IV.27   TFTTT

A   Above a Reynolds number of 2000, flow is likely to be turbulent.

B   Critical velocity depends also on the characteristics of the tube.

C,D   Laminar flow is more likely with a less dense (for example, helium) or a more viscous (for example, oil) fluid. The physicist regards both gases and liquids as fluids.

IV.28   FTTFT

A   These figures are much too high. 10 mA is somewhat higher than the 'let go' current, that is, the current at which direct stimulation of muscles prevents voluntary relaxation. 100 mA is a severe shock. Electric current becomes perceptible at about 0.2 mA and is objectionable by 1 mA.

D   Lower current is needed because the skin resistance is by-passed.

IV.29   TFFTF

B,C,D   The solubility is defined by the solubility coefficient and depends directly on the partial pressure (which, at a given temperature, is Henry's law). The partition coefficient describes the partition of a solute between two non-mixing solvents (and is most familiar to anaesthetists as the blood/gas coefficient of inhalational agents).

E   The Fick principle is used in indicator dilution techniques of calculating flow.

IV.30 FTTTT

A   Heat is the energy; temperature is the thermal *state* and is analogous to activity. The direction of net heat flow depends on the relative temperatures of two bodies not the total quantity of heat. (Consider a red-hot pin dropped into a bucket of boiling water.)

B   Resistance wire in a suitable electrical circuit can measure differences as small as 10^{-4}°C

D   The Seebeck effect is a temperature-sensitive voltage at the contact of two dissimilar metals.

Base excess
metabolic component
if uncomp = 0

$$HCO_3^- : H_2CO_3$$

$$20 : 1$$

plasma

Paper V   Questions

V.1 **Movement of water and solute between compartments in vivo may be by:**
- A solvent drag
- B filtration
- C osmosis
- D pinocytosis
- E diffusion.

V.2 **In an uncompensated respiratory alkalosis:**
- A the patient will be hypoventilating
- B the base excess may exceed 10 mmol/l
- C the arterial pH may be 7.65 or above
- D the concentration of ionised calcium in the plasma is decreased
- E the patient may show signs of tetanus.

V.3 **The following are true of buffer mechanisms:**
- A they protect the body against changes in pH until respiratory compensation occurs
- B quantitatively, haemoglobin is more important than plasma proteins as an extracellular buffer
- C ammonium excretion in a chronic acidosis permits conservation of bicarbonate
- D the normal ratio of concentrations of unionised to ionised in the carbonic acid/bicarbonate system is 20:1
- E plasma proteins are a relatively unimportant buffer mechanism in man.

V.4 **The tricarboxylic acid cycle:**
- A is the main mechanism of anaerobic glycolysis
- B has lipid as its main substrate
- C yields lactate as its main metabolite
- D generates four molecules of ATP per pyruvate molecule
- E generates four molecules of carbon dioxide per pyruvate molecule.

V.5 **The coronary blood flow:**
- A is about 500 ml/min at rest
- B supplies muscle that takes up 40 ml oxygen per minute at rest
- C is altered directly by vagal activity
- D ceases in systole
- E is autoregulated.

V.6 **The following are true of calcium balance:**

A   vitamin D stimulates calcium reabsorption from gut, bones and renal tubules

B   parathormone increases serum calcium

C   calcitonin decreases serum calcium

D   calcium absorption is reduced by steroids

E   calcium is excreted only in urine.

V.7 **Antidiuretic hormone (vasopressin):**

A   acts in the kidney by decreasing the permeability of certain membranes to water

B   induces smooth muscle contraction

C   has a biological half-life of 2 min

D   acts via cyclic AMP

E   is stored as neurophysin in the posterior pituitary.

V.8 **In the blood:**

A   basophils account for less than 0.5% of the total white count

B   megakaryocytes break up to form platelets

C   globulins are the commonest type of protein

D   most lymphocytes are of extramedullary origin

E   opsonisation facilitates phagocytosis by lymphocytes.

V.9 **The knee jerk:**

A   is a monosynaptic reflex

B   arises from the spinal cord at T12

C   has afferents within the quadriceps tendon

D   is modified by output from higher centres

E   has a reaction time of about 20 ms.

V.10 **In the physiology of vision:**

A   colour vision is restricted to the optic disc

B   colour blindness is about 15 times commoner in men than women

C   all colours of the spectrum can be produced by mixing the basic colours red, yellow and blue

D   the ultra-violet region has a longer wavelength than visible light

E   the rods are more sensitive to light than the cones.

V.11 The following hormones are produced in important amounts by the adrenal cortex:
- A androgens
- B glucocorticoids
- C corticotrophin (ACTH)
- D aldosterone
- E erythropoietin.

V.12 In a fit 30-year-old male:
- A the alveolar ventilation at rest is 4.2 l/min
- B the maximum voluntary ventilation is 125–170 l/min
- C the functional residual capacity is 1.2 litres
- D intrapleural pressure decreases to – 30 cmH$_2$O at maximum inspiration
- E the normal ventilatory rate is 12–15 breaths per minute.

V.13 Breathing even very low concentrations of carbon monoxide is dangerous because:
- A carbon monoxide has a high affinity for reduced haemoglobin
- B blood can be completely saturated with carbon monoxide at a partial pressure of 0.66 kPa (5 mmHg)
- C carbon monoxide is extremely soluble in plasma
- D carboxyhaemoglobin dissociation is irreversible within 2 h
- E carboxyhaemoglobin alters red cell shape leading to aggregation.

V.14 Hypoxic hypoxia:
- A is caused by defective pulmonary oxygen transfer
- B is caused by a reduction in inspired PO_2
- C occurs in severe anaemia
- D is caused by depression of the respiratory centre
- E is exacerbated by hypothermia.

V.15 Erythromycin:
- A is a suitable alternative for patients who are allergic to penicillin
- B is contraindicated in pregnancy
- C is used in atypical pneumonia
- D is mainly excreted unchanged in the urine
- E should be given by rapid injection rather than slow infusion.

V.16 Dopexamine hydrochloride:
- A is a β_1-agonist
- B inhibits neuronal uptake of noradrenaline
- C is an agonist at dopaminergic receptors
- D causes splanchnic vasoconstriction
- E is contraindicated in patients with aortic stenosis.

V.17 Atropine:

  A   inhibits sweating
  B   crosses the placental barrier
  C   has local anaesthetic properties
  D   is totally metabolised in the liver
  E   increases tone in the internal laryngeal muscles.

V.18 Amiodarone:

  A   prolongs the cardiac action potential
  B   is mainly excreted in the urine
  C   may cause heart block when a general anaesthetic is given
  D   may alter the effects of anticoagulants
  E   may alter the appearance of computerised tomography (CT)
      scans.

V.19 A metabolic alkalosis inhibits the diuretic action of:

  A   spironolactone
  B   chlorothiazide
  C   acetazolamide
  D   mersalyl
  E   frusemide.

**V.20 The hypoglycaemic effect of the sulphonylureas is reduced
by:**

  A   propranolol
  B   phenylbutazone
  C   intravenous calcium gluconate
  D   the oral contraceptives
  E   bendrofluazide.

V.21 Nitrous oxide:

  A   is produced commercially by heating ammonium nitrate to
      240°C
  B   gas is stored in metal cylinders at 51 atmospheres
  C   as available for medical use may contain small amounts of
      nitric oxide and nitrogen dioxide
  D   is 15 times more soluble than oxygen in blood
  E   has a blood/gas partition coefficient of 0.47.

V.22 Ketamine:

  A   is a potent analgesic
  B   is rapidly metabolised in the liver
  C   releases noradrenaline
  D   produces muscular relaxation
  E   does not depress the cardiovascular system.

V.23 Morphine is metabolised by:

  A conjugation with a glucuronide
  B monoamine oxidase
  C acetylation
  D esterases in the blood stream
  E hydrolysis.

V.24 Carbonic anhydrase:

  A catalyses the formation of carbonic acid from carbon dioxide
  B is present in greater quantities in the gastric oxyntic cells
     than in the red blood cells
  C increases the production of aqueous humour
  D inhibitors affect renal tubular function
  E inhibitors produce respiratory depression.

V.25 These drugs interact with plasma cholinesterase:

  A nitrogen mustard
  B suxamethonium
  C procaine
  D ecothiopate
  E trimetaphan.

V.26 Pethidine:

  A increases cerebrospinal fluid pressure
  B is a local analgesic
  C produces vasoconstriction
  D has anti-spasmodic properties
  E has an anticholinergic action.

V.27 When measuring central venous pressure:

  A a catheter should not be advanced further than 20 cm in any
     patient
  B the diameter of the catheter should not exceed 0.25 mm
  C the subclavian route may be used
  D the zero point should be taken from the sternal angle even
     when the patient is sitting up
  E a dependent loop of tubing should be avoided to prevent
     back flow of blood into the catheter.

V.28   The following statements are true:

    A   carbon monoxide is used in the measurement of functional residual capacity

    B   the measurement of pulmonary gas transfer factor necessitates the use of an inert gas such as helium

    C   the normal FEV_1:FVC ratio should be in excess of 75% in a 50-year-old man

    D   0.3 ml oxygen per 100 ml blood are dissolved when breathing room air and with a haemoglobin of 15 gm/dl

    E   approximately 72% of the blood volume is contained within the normal venous circulation.

V.29   An automated oscillotonometric blood pressure monitor (for example, a Dinamap®):

    A   calculates mean arterial pressure from measurement of systolic and diastolic pressure

    B   is more accurate at measuring systolic than diastolic pressure

    C   will take more time to measure blood pressure if heart rate is slower

    D   performs better than an arterial line in patients in atrial fibrillation

    E   tends to overread low blood pressures.

V.30   When a liquid boils:

    A   its vapour pressure is 101 kPa

    B   its latent heat of vaporisation is zero

    C   bubbles of vapour form on irregularities in the container

    D   the temperature of the liquid cannot exceed the boiling point

    E   it will contain little or no dissolved gas.

Paper V   Answers

V.1   TTTTT
These are all correct.

V.2   FFTTF

A   By definition, a respiratory alkalosis is caused by hyperventilation.
B   If uncompensated, the base excess (metabolic component) will be zero.
E   You are unlikely to meet a question like this in the actual exam; it is here merely to stress the importance of reading the question — it should, of course, read 'tetany' and the answer would then be 'true'.

V.3   FTTFT

A   Respiratory changes and buffer mechanisms are interlinked, although you can consider buffering as a phenomenon that could take place, independently of physiology, in a test tube. Re-equilibrium is established through renal compensation if the acid-base disturbance is respiratory.
D   This is the correct ratio but it is the wrong way round: ionised:unionised is 20:1.
E   Beware of considering **B** and **E** together, taking **B** as true and therefore **E** as false; plasma proteins are important buffers.

V.4   FFFFT

A   The tricarboxylic acid cycle is the mechanism of *aerobic* metabolism.
B   The immediate substrate is pyruvate, most of which is generated from carbohydrates.
C   Carbon dioxide and hydrogen ions are the main products.
D   ATP is generated from NADH outside the cycle.

V.5   FTFFT

A   Coronary blood flow at rest is 250 ml/min.
C   The question says 'directly'. The vagus alters coronary blood flow only indirectly, by its negative inotropic effect.
D   Two-thirds of coronary blood flow occurs during diastole, and one-third during systole. There is no *subendocardial* flow during systole.

V.6   TTTTF

D   Steroids depress vitamin D stimulation of calcium absorption.

E   Calcium is excreted mainly by secretion into the gut.

V.7   FTFTF

A   Membrane permeability is *increased* via V_2 receptors in the tubular cells of the loop of Henle and collecting duct.

B   Vasopressin causes vascular constriction amongst other actions.

C   The biological half-life is 18 min.

E   Neurophysin is stored with vasopressin in the Herring bodies of the posterior pituitary, but it is discarded parts of the precursor molecules.

V.8   TFFTF

A   Basophils make up 0.4% of the white count.

B   Platelets are produced in the bone marrow, not the blood; take care to refer back to the stem when answering each branch.

C   Globulins make up about 40% of plasma proteins; albumin makes up 55%.

D   Most lymphocytes are formed in the lymph nodes, thymus and spleen.

E   Opsonisation is the process by which complement binds to bacteria, which are then more easily destroyed by the neutrophil granulocytes.

V.9   TFFTT

A,B   The knee jerk is an example of the stretch reflex, the only monosynaptic reflex. The spinal level is L3–4.

C   The afferents are the muscle spindles within the muscle. The receptors in the tendons are the Golgi tendon organs that subserve the inverse stretch reflex, a bisynaptic reflex.

E   This monosynaptic reflex is very rapid.

V.10   FTFFT

A   The optic disc has no receptors; it is the blind spot. The fovea contains only cones, but cones are not restricted to this part of the retina.

B   Colour blindness occurs in 0.5% women and 9% men.

C   The three colours for colour addition (that is, using light) are red, green and violet.

D   Ultra-violet is the shorter wavelengths, less than about 400 nm.

E   The rods have greater sensitivity; the cones have greater acuity.

V.11 TTFTF

C Corticotrophin (ACTH) is produced in the anterior pituitary and controls release of adrenal cortical hormones.

E 90% of erythropoietin is produced in the kidney glomeruli, the rest in the liver.

V.12 TTFTT

C The residual volume is 1.2 litres; the FRC is 2.2 litres.

E A simple question.

V.13 TTFFF

A,B Death occurs when 70–80% haemoglobin is combined as carboxyhaemoglobin.

C Carbon monoxide is not especially soluble in plasma.

D The combination of carbon monoxide with haemoglobin is fully reversible as soon as the victim is removed from the poisonous atmosphere. Dissociation is speeded by higher concentrations of oxygen.

E Alteration of the shape of the red cell is what happens in sickling.

V.14 TTFTF

Hypoxic hypoxia occurs when the availability of oxygen to the red blood cell from the atmosphere is decreased.

C This is anaemic hypoxia.

E Hypothermia shifts the oxyhaemoglobin dissociation curve to the left, reducing oxygen delivery and maintaining arterial oxygen content. Hypothermia also reduces oxygen utilisation and demand.

V.15 TFTFF

B There is no evidence that erythromycin is hazardous in pregnancy.

D It is mainly excreted in the liver.

E Erythromycin is irritant and must be well diluted and infused slowly.

V.16 FTTFT

A Dopexamine is a β_2-agonist.

D It causes splanchnic vasodilation, which may improve blood flow to gut mucosa in shocked patients.

E It is an inotrope and peripheral vasodilator. Vasodilation can be dangerous in patients with left ventricular outflow obstruction.

V.17 TTTFF
  D   Enzymatic hydrolysis occurs in other tissues as well as in the liver.
  E   Atropine has no effect on the laryngeal muscles.

V.18 TFTTT
  A   Amiodarone is a Class 3 agent.
  B   It is mostly excreted in bile and faeces; less than 5% is excreted by the kidneys.
  C   This is in the data sheet produced by the manufacturer.
  D   The dose of warfarin may need adjustment.
  E   Amiodarone contains iodine, which is radio-opaque on scan.

V.19 FFFTF
  A   Spironolactone is an aldosterone antagonist.
  C   Acetazolamide is a carbonic anhydrase inhibitor used to treat metabolic alkalosis. Its more well-known use is in the prophylaxis of altitude sickness.
  D   Mersalyl is a mercury diuretic. Mercury diuretics are no longer used (so do not worry if you had not heard of mersalyl) but they are useful in discussions of diuretic action. Excess loss of chloride over bicarbonate produces a metabolic alkalosis and the mercurous ion is not converted to the active mercuric form.

V.20 FFFTT
  Always be wary if a diabetic on oral hypoglycaemics is on other drugs. The hypoglycaemic effect may be enhanced by, amongst others, β-blockers (**A**) and agents that are strongly protein-bound (**B**). β-blockers also mask the symptoms and signs of hypoglycaemia.
  C   A red herring: calcium has no known important effect either way.

V.21 TTFTT
  C   These theoretical contaminants are highly toxic.

V.22 TTTFT
  D   Ketamine increases tone.

V.23 TFFFF

Most morphine is eventually excreted in the urine, although 10% may appear in the faeces. In animals some is metabolised by N-demethylation but this degradation pathway has not been shown in man.

V.24 TTTTF

B　There is 5–6 times as much carbonic anhydrase in gastric cells.

D　Although almost 99% inhibition must be present for this to be important.

E　Inhibition leads to carbon dioxide accumulation and therefore to respiratory *stimulation*.

V.25 FTTTT

A　Nitrogen mustard is a corrosive agent, and related to some anti-cancer drugs; it is the organophosphorus poison gases that interfere with cholinesterase.

V.26 TTFTT

C　Pethidine causes mild vasodilation and also has a quinidine-like effect, which cause a decrease in blood pressure.

V.27 FFTFF

A　This might be true for a catheter inserted centrally, but not if insertion is from the antecubital fossa.

B　Read carefully: a quarter of a millimetre!

D　You should be able to discuss the details of the measurement of the CVP and the merits and accuracy of the various sites taken as zero.

E　A dependent loop lessens the risk of air embolus.

V.28   FFTTT

A,B   Helium dilution is used to measure the FRC; carbon
monoxide to estimate the transfer factor.

V.29   FTTFT

A   Some early auscultatory monitors did this, but
oscillotonometers measure mean arterial pressure as the
point of maximum oscillation in the cuff.

D   It may be difficult or impossible to obtain an accurate
measure of blood pressure in patients with atrial fibrillation
(systolic blood pressure fluctuates beat-to-beat).

E   Most non-invasive monitors have a flattened response
compared with invasive arterial monitoring.

V.30   FFTFT

A   The vapour pressure will equal the ambient pressure,
which may be 101 kPa but depends on altitude and
prevailing conditions.

B   The energy for vaporisation has to be supplied for the
liquid to keep boiling. Only at the critical temperature does
the latent heat become zero.

C   Bubbles also form on particles in the liquid.

D   Liquids can be 'superheated'.

Paper VI Questions

VI.1 Alpha-adrenergic stimulation produces:
  A vasodilation
  B tachycardia
  C uterine relaxation in pregnancy
  D a positive inotropic effect
  E intestinal relaxation.

VI.2 In human nutrition:
  A the basic energy requirement for a 70 kg man is about 8400 kJ (2000 kcal)
  B carbohydrates are the most compact energy source
  C the respiratory quotient (RQ) decreases when fat is the main energy source being utilised
  D essential amino acids are those which participate in metabolic reactions
  E a high protein diet raises the metabolic rate.

VI.3 In an isolated nerve-muscle preparation, for instance the sciatic nerve and gastrocnemius muscle taken from a frog:
  A passive stretch causes an approximately linear increase in tension
  B active tension is greatest at the anatomical resting length of the muscle
  C velocity of contraction decreases with increasing load on the muscle
  D tetanic stimulation increases active tension at a given muscle length
  E isotonic force is measured by fixing both ends of the muscle.

VI.4 The QRS deflection on the electrocardiogram:
  A is normally longer than 0.2 s
  B is caused by ventricular repolarisation
  C is prolonged in bundle branch block
  D represents the phase of isovolumetric contraction
  E is absent in complete block of atrioventricular conduction.

VI.5 Synapses:
  A in mammalian nerve have synaptic clefts about 20 nm wide
  B in the CNS are mainly in white matter
  C permit conduction in only one direction
  D are absent in the parasympathetic ganglia
  E are present in the dorsal root ganglia.

VI.6   Angiotensin II:

A   acts directly on vascular smooth muscle rather than via
α-receptors

B   is formed in the lungs

C   is an octapeptide

D   is synthesised from angiotensin I by the same enzyme that
breaks down bradykinin

E   concentrations are decreased when a subject stands after a
period of sitting.

VI.7   In exercise:

A   oxygen consumption increases in proportion to lactate
production

B   mixed venous oxygen tension decreases

C   blood flow increases to all organs except the brain

D   the number of patent capillaries in skeletal muscle increases

E   systemic blood flow rises more rapidly than pulmonary
blood flow.

**VI.8   The anticoagulant effect of a massive blood transfusion
may be due to:**

A   deficient factor V and VIII

B   inactive platelets

C   increased circulating tissue plasminogen activator

D   cold

E   vitamin K availability.

VI.9   The concentration gradient in the renal medulla:

A   is generated in equal part by each nephron

B   is independent of urine flow

C   depends on active transport of sodium

D   depends on urea maintaining the high osmolality in the
pyramids

E   can be maintained by aerobic or anaerobic metabolism.

**VI.10   Amongst the features of acclimatisation to high altitude
are:**

A   an increase in oxygen-carrying capacity

B   an increase in respiratory minute volume

C   an increase in cardiac output

D   a compensatory decrease in heart rate

E   redistribution of blood flow away from the pulmonary
vascular bed.

VI.11 Hypercapnia:
- A causes sweating
- B increases parasympathetic activity
- C depresses ventilation if extreme
- D has a direct positive inotropic action
- E aids the uptake of oxygen in the lung.

VI.12 Apart from that carried in simple solution, carbon dioxide is carried in the blood:
- A in the red cells
- B as buffered carbonic acid
- C in direct combination with oxyhaemoglobin
- D as phosphate esters
- E combined with plasma proteins.

VI.13 Noradrenaline depletion is produced by:
- A reserpine
- B phentolamine
- C trimetaphan
- D guanethidine
- E hydralazine.

VI.14 Propranolol:
- A decreases cardiac output
- B causes tachycardia
- C causes bradycardia
- D decreases secretion of renin
- E is useful in the treatment of heart failure.

VI.15 Midazolam:
- A is water-soluble
- B accumulates in body fat
- C rarely causes venous thrombosis
- D should not be given a second time within 2 weeks
- E may induce epileptiform EEG changes.

VI.16 Sodium nitroprusside:
    A   affects both resistance and capacitance vessels
    B   reduces renal blood flow
    C   is metabolised to ferrocyanide
    D   should be made up for infusion in 5% dextrose
    E   is contraindicated for treatment of the hypertension of aortic
          coarctation.

VI.17 Intravenous induction agents:
    A   must be water-soluble
    B   are taken up preferentially by the reticular activating system
    C   cross the placental barrier
    D   reduce the velocity of axonal transmission in myelinated
          fibres
    E   cause agent-specific EEG changes.

VI.18 Competitive antagonism:
    A   usually refers to competition with enzymes at the site of
          action of the drug
    B   causes a rightward shift of the dose–response curve
    C   is true of the competition of cyanides for the cytochrome
          system
    D   is true of β-adrenergic blockers and sympathomimetic
          amines
    E   is possible only if the receptors are fully occupied.

VI.19 The following drugs have antihistaminic activity:
    A   promethazine
    B   ranitidine
    C   cyclizine
    D   mepyramine
    E   chlorpheniramine.

VI.20 Ropivacaine:
    A   is an ester-linked local anaesthetic
    B   is a chiral drug
    C   has a duration of action similar to lignocaine at equipotent
          doses
    D   is a vasoconstrictor at clinical concentrations
    E   may cause convulsions.

VI.21 The actions of non-depolarising neuromuscular blocking drugs:

A   are potentiated by anaesthetic vapours
B   when given in repeated doses can be described as dual block
C   are potentiated by intraperitoneal tobramycin
D   are potentiated in patients with multiple neurofibromatosis
E   are potentiated in hyperkalaemia.

VI.22 The following have interactions likely to be of clinical importance:

A   terfenadine and antibiotics
B   prednisolone and carbenoxolone
C   insulin and phenoxybenzamine
D   alcohol and warfarin
E   labetalol and ranitidine.

VI.23 The following are true of these biological potentials:

A   the potentials in the EEG are approximately 50 μV
B   the beta waves of the EEG are of 15–60 Hz range
C   the alpha waves of the EEG are of 70–100 Hz range
D   the patient is not at risk from electrocution during recording of the EEG because of the small potentials
E   the electromyogram is unlikely to interfere with the EEG because of the difference in electrical potential.

VI.24 If an anaesthetic machine calibrated for sea level is moved to high altitude:

A   the flowmeter bobbins will underread the gas flow
B   the anaesthetic vapours will boil at a lower temperature
C   nitrous oxide cylinders will expand
D   the pitch of the oxygen alarm will be different from pitch at sea level
E   a higher inspired oxygen concentration will be required to maintain oxygen saturation in the patient.

VI.25   Non-parametric tests:

A   can apply to samples that are not distributed normally

B   can be used on small samples

C   are generally mathematically easier than parametric tests

D   imply that the variable cannot be measured accurately

E   an example is the Wilcoxon matched-pairs signed-rank test.

VI.26   The following are true of electromagnetic radiation:

A   it includes visible light

B   infra-red radiation occurs only from objects that are hotter than the environment

C   the Stefan–Boltzmann law defines the heat radiated from a black body

D   it obeys the inverse square law

E   it includes ultrasound.

VI.27   The following need to be known to calculate the volume of vapour obtained at STP from the complete evaporation of a liquid:

A   the saturated vapour pressure of the liquid

B   Avogadro's number

C   the liquid density

D   the molecular weight

E   the volume of liquid.

VI.28   In the measurement of carbon dioxide:

A   the Lloyd–Haldane apparatus measures carbon dioxide by chemical methods

B   infra-red absorption can be used

C   carbon dioxide absorbs light at a wavelength of 430 nm

D   carbon monoxide may interfere

E   carbon dioxide cannot be distinguished from nitrous oxide with a mass spectrometer.

VI.29   In a consideration of osmosis:

A   osmolarity is milliosmoles per litre of water

B   osmolality is milliosmoles per litre of a specific solvent

C   the depression of freezing point of a solution is inversely proportional to its osmolality

D   the depression of vapour pressure of a solvent is proportional to the molar concentration of the solute

E   there are osmometers that depend on the principle of depression of vapour pressure.

VI.30 **The sine function:**

    A is the pattern of alternating current (AC)
    B describes the motion of a freely-moving pendulum
    C has a maximum value of 1 and a minimum of 0
    D is a hyperbolic function
    E is the natural logarithm of the cosine.

Paper VI Answers

VI.1 **FFFFT**

A α-agonists cause vasoconstriction.

B There is reflex bradycardia secondary to increased peripheral resistance. There is no direct chronotropic effect.

C Noradrenaline *increases* the tone of the pregnant uterus.

D α-adrenergic stimulation has no inotropic effect.

E There is intestinal relaxation, but gastrointestinal sphincteric tone is also increased.

VI.2 **TFTFT**

B Fats yield about 39 kJ (9.3 kcal) per gram, compared with 17.2 kj (4.1 kcal) for carbohydrate.

C RQ for carbohydrate is 1; for fats is 0.7.

D Essential amino acids are those that the body cannot produce in sufficient quantities.

E A protein diet raises metabolic rate by 15–20%: the 'specific dynamic action'.

VI.3 **TTTTF**

A Tension increases linearly (Hooke's law) until eventually the muscle fibres tear.

E Iso*metric* force is measured by fixing both ends of the muscle.

VI.4 **FFTFF**

A The QRS is 0.08–0.10 s.

B The QRS is ventricular *de*polarisation; the T wave is *re*polarisation.

C The QRS is particularly prolonged in left bundle branch block.

D The phase of isovolumetric contraction ends when the tricuspid and mitral valves open. The QRS marks the beginning of this phase, but cannot represent it: one is an electrical event, the other a mechanical one.

E Complexes will be abnormal, but absence would cause Stokes–Adams attacks or death.

VI.5 **TFTFT**

B The white matter is mainly axons; the grey matter cell bodies and synapses.

D Parasympathetic ganglia are the junction between pre- and postganglionic nerve fibres and, as with all other neuronal links, there are synapses.

VI.6 **TTTTF**

B 70% of angiotensin I is converted to angiotensin II during a single passage through the lung. This conversion also occurs in other tissues.

D The enzyme is peptidyl dipeptidase. Captopril, used in the treatment of hypertension, inhibits this enzyme and thus blocks the synthesis of both the most active vasoconstrictor known (angiotensin II) and the breakdown of the potent vasodilator, bradykinin.

VI.7 **FTFTF**

A Both oxygen consumption and lactate production increase, but not in proportion to each other.

C Blood flow to the splanchnic bed and liver may be 20% of resting levels.

E Impossible! Think about it.

VI.8 **TTTTF**

C tPa may be released as an effect of increased circulating catecholamines and vasopressin. The drug aprotinin counteracts this response and reduces blood loss.

D Cold may cause abnormal agglutination in susceptible patients. More importantly, hypothermia slows down enzymatic reactions and delays clotting.

E There are long-term stores of vitamin K and acute deficiency does not occur.

VI.9 **FFTTF**

A Not all the loops are of equal length.

B Very high flow can wash solutes out of the medulla.

C,E The active transport of sodium is energy-dependent and requires aerobic metabolism.

VI.10 **TTTFF**

A Polycythaemia increases oxygen-carrying capacity.

C The increase in cardiac output is less important than the changes in respiration, except at very high altitude.

D There is tachycardia.

VI.11 TTTFF

B Hypercapnia increases parasympathetic activity but the effects are overshadowed by concurrent sympathetic activity.

D Carbon dioxide is a negative inotrope. Its indirect effects via the sympathetic nervous system and catecholamine secretion are positively inotropic.

E The dissociation curve moves to the right, oxygen affinity is decreased and thus it is release in the tissues that is facilitated.

VI.12 TTFFF

C Carbon dioxide combines with reduced haemoglobin.

VI.13 TFFTF

A Reserpine is now rarely used but because of its actions is an important drug in theoretical pharmacology; it depletes stores of catecholamines and 5-HT in many organs.

B Phentolamine is an α-adrenergic blocker.

C Trimetaphan is a post-synaptic competitive inhibitor of acetylcholine at both sympathetic and parasympathetic ganglia.

D Guanethidine depletes noradrenaline stores in spleen, heart and blood vessels.

E Hydralazine is a direct acting vasodilator.

VI.14 TFTTF

B,C Though not true of propranolol, there are drugs that can cause either bradycardia or tachycardia, for example, atropine.

D Propranolol is particularly useful in hypertension in which there are high renin levels.

E It is a negative inotrope and makes heart failure worse, though would indirectly treat heart failure secondary to a supraventricular tachycardia.

VI.15 TTTFF

D There is no evidence for this.

E The benzodiazepines are anti-convulsants.

VI.16   TFFTT

B   In hypotension caused by hypovolaemia, renal blood flow is reduced by vasoconstriction; the hypotension caused by SNP (used appropriately) occurs with vasodilatation, and renal blood flow is not compromised.

C   Ferrocyanide is not formed at all, either as a result of body metabolism or therapeutic intervention. In the treatment of cyanide poisoning, cyanide ions and thiosulphate form *thiocyanate*.

VI.17   FFTFT

A   Propofol, for example, is not soluble in water; it is made soluble by emulsification.

B   The production of unconsciousness is presumed to be because of effects on the reticular activating system, but there is not preferential uptake.

D   The mode of action of anaesthetics is unknown, but is certainly not because of alteration of axonal transmission.

VI.18   FTFTF

A   Competitive antagonism refers to action at specific receptors that are usually components of cell membranes.

B   At low drug concentrations, non-competitive antagonism has the same effect.

C   Cyanide chelates the metallic moiety of cytochrome oxidase irreversibly.

E   Competitive antagonism can be recognised only if there is some activity at the receptors, but that does not require full occupancy.

VI.19   TTTTT

Many drugs that are not antihistamines have antihistaminic properties.

VI.20   FFFTT

A   Ropivacaine is amide-linked.

B   Chiral drugs are stereoisomeric mixtures. The parent compound (N-alkyl pipecholyl xylidine) exists in S and R forms, but ropivacaine is the S-isomer.

C   Duration of action is similar to bupivacaine.

D   Ropivacaine is a vasoconstrictor over a wide range of concentrations.

VI.21 TFTTF

B   Dual block is a confusing term, which some use to mean the phase II block that occurs with prolonged administration of depolarising agents. As dual block is a term derived from observations made in particular animal experiments, it is best not used.

E   Hyperkalaemia may be precipitated by suxamethonium but does not alter the response to non-depolarisers.

VI.22 TTFTF

A   This combination may cause QT prolongation and lead to arrhythmias, including *torsades de pointes*. Ketoconazole and erythromycin are the main antibiotics implicated.

B   Prednisolone and carbenoxolone may cause potassium loss.

C   No: the interaction of insulin is with β-blockers.

D   Alcohol can inhibit liver enzymes, reducing the requirement for warfarin.

E   Cimetidine, but not ranitidine, increases the metabolism of β-blockers.

VI.23 TTFFF

C   These figures are too large. The alpha waves are of 7–10 Hz range, smaller than the beta waves.

D   Any accident would be caused by a fault in the measuring instrument, with the current coming from outside the body; the potential being measured is irrelevant.

E   The potentials overlap considerably: the EMG is 10–80 μV.

VI.24 FTTTT

A   The actual flow of gas through a bobbin flowmeter at altitude is greater than indicated because the gas density is reduced. The error is about 1% per 300 m rise in altitude.

B   Clinically, the increased delivery of vapour compensates for the need to provide a greater inspired concentration to maintain the same partial pressure of vapour within the patient.

C   Because external pressure is less, the pressure across the cylinder wall increases.

E   The requirement for increased inspired oxygen makes nitrous oxide anaesthesia impractical as it is impossible to give the gas at a high enough partial pressure.

VI.25   TTTFT

   D   Non-parametric tests make no assumption about the
           accuracy of the observed variable.

VI.26   TFTTF

   B   There may be no net transfer of heat but that does not
           mean that there is no infra-red radiation.
   C   The Stefan–Boltzmann Law states that the rate of
           emission of heat from a black body is proportional to the
           fourth power of its absolute temperature.
   E   Ultrasound is, as the name implies, sound energy.

VI.27   FFTTT

   A   The saturated vapour pressure will tell something of the
           rate of evaporation but not the volume.
   B   Avogadro's number is the number of particles in a mole of
           a substance (6.022×10^{23}).

VI.28   TTTFF

   A   The Lloyd–Haldane apparatus is a laboratory standard, but
           is not in clinical use.
   D   *Nitrous oxide* may interfere.
   E   Carbon dioxide and nitrous oxide have the same mass
           number (44) but the gases can be separated by
           identification of fragments produced by ionisation, for
           example, nitric oxide (NO).

VI.29   FFFTT

   A,B Osmola*R*ity is per lit*R*e; osmola*L*ity is per ki*L*ogram. In
            anaesthesia, the solvent is usually water, but the general
            definition must be per litre (or kilogram) of *solvent*.
   C   Depression of freezing point of a solution is *directly*
            proportional to its osmolality: needs clear thinking!
   D   This is Raoult's law.

VI.30 TTFFF

C   The sine function is symmetrical around a mean of zero: maximum is + 1 and minimum is − 1.

D   It is what it is: a sine function. It is an example of a trigonometric function.

E   The sine is the inverse of the cosine.

Paper VII Questions

VII.1 ✓ **Bicarbonate:**

    A in the renal tubular cell does not normally require carbonic anhydrase for production

    B concentration in cells is 10–20 mmol/l

    C concentration in plasma is 25 mmol/l

    D occupies a 'volume' that is about one-third body weight

    E concentrations increase in potassium depletion.

VII.2 ✓ **In cellular metabolism:**

    A the Krebs cycle is obligatorily aerobic

    B one molecule of glucose can yield 38 molecules of adenosine triphosphate (ATP)

    C the aerobic oxidation of glucose is 100% efficient

    D oxidative phosphorylation occurs in the mitochondrion

    E carbohydrates have a lower respiratory quotient than fats.

VII.3 ✓ **In the control of cardiac output in normal man the following are true:**

    A alteration of heart rate is an intrinsic response

    B beat-by-beat left ventricular output equals beat-by-beat right ventricular output

    C heart rate increases before stroke volume in exercise

    D an increase in ventricular filling pressure decreases stroke volume

    E cardiac output increases in fever.

VII.4 **The following are true of phosphate:**

    A 85% of total body phosphate is in bone

    B normal plasma phosphate is 0.2–0.7 mmol/l

    C serum phosphate concentrations are increased by parathormone

    D phosphate is an important intracellular buffer

    E phosphate is important in the formation of high energy nucleotides.

leu chen

VII.5 Of the opioid peptides:

A endorphins are short-chain peptides   *pentapeptide.*
B enkephalins are short-chain peptides
C enkephalins are exclusive to the central nervous system
D β-endorphin is secreted by the pituitary gland
E the natural ligand for the μ-receptor is substance P.

VII.6 Erythropoietin:

A production is increased by hypoxia
B produces a measurable rise in red cell mass within 6 h
C is produced partly in the liver
D production is facilitated by catecholamines
E is inactivated in the liver.

VII.7 The velocity of impulse propagation along nerve fibres:

A increases with diameter in myelinated fibres
B is independent of diameter in unmyelinated fibres
C is altered in hypokalaemia
D is unaffected by tetanic stimulation
E has no clinical application.

VII.8 The effects of cortisol on the kidney include:

A increased free water clearance
B decreased sodium reabsorption
C increased glomerular filtration rate
D an indirect increase of the water permeability of the collecting duct
E increased glucose reabsorption.

unmyelinated velocity $\propto \sqrt{D}$

myelinated velocity $\propto D$

VII.9 In a consideration of pulmonary gas exchange, the following are true:

    A the area of the alveolar membrane is effectively 70 m^2
    B pulmonary capillaries have the same diameter as red cells
    C the alveolar capillary membrane is two cells thick
    D there is countercurrent flow between alveolar gas and capillary blood
    E there are ligand-gated channels for oxygen transfer.

VII.10 **During moderate exercise:**

    A the diffusion distance for oxygen in skeletal muscle is decreased
    B there is selective streaming of red cells to muscle capillaries
    C arterial haemoglobin saturation is unaffected
    D arterial carbon dioxide tension increases
    E the respiratory quotient becomes higher.

VII.11 **Cell wall synthesis is the primary site of action of:**

    A chloramphenicol
    B penicillin
    C sulphonamides
    D tetracyclines
    E aminoglycosides.

VII.12 **Hyoscine:**

    A is a central nervous system stimulant
    B is amnesic
    C is absorbed through the skin
    D induces bronchoconstriction
    E is effective in motion sickness.

VII.13 Carbamazepine:

A   is a first-line drug for glossopharyngeal neuralgia
B   induces drug-metabolising enzymes
C   causes fluid retention
D   causes a dry mouth
E   causes extrapyramidal symptoms in renal failure.

VII.14 Glyceryl trinitrate:

A   directly reduces myocardial oxygen consumption
B   dilates veins more than arteries
C   favours subendocardial perfusion
D   increases venous return
E   is effective prophylactically before exercise.

VII.15 The barbiturates:

A   are a family of compounds derived from malonic and uric acids
B   have decreased duration of action if more lipid soluble
C   were first used as induction agents in the First World War
D   may become convulsants with N-substitution
E   inhibit GABA-ergic transmission in experimental preparations.

VII.16 Isoflurane:

A   is a halogenated hydrocarbon
B   is metabolised very little in humans
C   depresses respiration less than enflurane
D   has a blood:gas solubility of 1.91
E   causes renal damage in high concentrations.

VII.17 Clinically significant amounts of the following drugs will cross the normal blood–brain barrier when given in the usual dosage:

A   streptomycin
B   sulphadimidine
C   benzyl penicillin
D   tubocurarine
E   diazepam.

VII.18 Proteinase inhibitors include:

A   streptokinase
B   tranexamic acid
C   plasmin
D   aprotinin
E   epsilon amino caproic acid.

VII.19 Desflurane:

A   has a blood/gas partition coefficient lower than nitrous oxide

B   has a minimal alveolar concentration approximately the same as enflurane

C   has a high boiling point

D   can be used with soda-lime

E   allows rapid emergence from anaesthesia.

VII.20 Nalbuphine:

A   is an agonist–antagonist opioid

B   depresses ventilation less than an equianalgesic dose of morphine

C   may precipitate withdrawal in morphine dependency

D   has dysphoric side-effects

E   has less abuse potential than morphine.

VII.21 Neostigmine:

A   has no effect presynaptically at the neuromuscular junction

B   has little effect at muscarinic cholinoceptors

C   can cause bronchospasm

D   is active by mouth

E   is partly broken down by pseudocholinesterase.

VII.22 The following are true for pulse oximeters:

A   they incorporate LEDs (light-emitting diodes)

B   the wavelengths are in the infra-red and ultra-violet

C   only changes in arterial blood are sensed

D   they measure absorption at the isobestic point

E   they are reliable in methaemoglobinaemia.

VII.23 An end-tidal sample of expired air from a normal adult:

A   has a content of carbon dioxide of approximately 5%

B   approximates to alveolar gas

C   more closely corresponds to the arterial partial pressure of carbon dioxide if the preceding inspiration was maximal

D   has a water content of about 6%

E   will tend to under-estimate the arterial partial pressure of carbon dioxide if tidal volumes are small.

VII.24 The following are true in a consideration of the measurement of acid-base balance:

A   a litre of pure water contains 10^{-7} g of H^+ ions

B   pK varies with temperature

C   pH is directly proportional to the logarithm of the carbon dioxide tension

D   the relation between pH and hydrogen ion concentration is approximately linear over the normal range of pH

E   a change of 1 pH unit is a 100-fold change in hydrogen ion concentration.

VII.25 The following are true of flow:

A   it is volume per unit time

B   laminar flow is about twice as fast in the centre of a tube as the overall mean flow

C   laminar flow is directly proportional to pressure difference

D   doubling the radius of a tube increases laminar flow by four times

E   turbulent flow is proportional to the square of the pressure difference.

VII.26 In a normal adult on the average diet, the following are excreted in the urine in 24 h:

A   150 mmol sodium

B   25 mmol potassium

C   10 mmol glucose

D   5 mmol calcium

E   25 mmol creatinine.

VII.27 In a consideration of electrical safety:

A   skin impedance is reduced when wet

B   potentials below 24 V AC are safe

C   the diathermy neutral plate must be connected directly to earth

D   5% dextrose does not conduct electricity

E   battery-operated equipment is safe.

VII.28 When recording an electrical signal:

A   mains interference is eliminated by isolating equipment from earth

B   electrical filters reduce the signal-to-noise ratio

C   the frequency response of a suitable recorder should be linear to about the 10th harmonic of the fundamental

D   matching of equipment impedances is important

E   zero stability may depend on temperature.

VII.29   **The following are true:**

A   work is force multiplied by distance
B   the joule is a unit of energy
C   power is the total work expended
D   mass and weight are related by gravity
E   the efficiency of a mechanical process is work-in related to work-out.

VII.30   **In a consideration of temperature and its measurement:**

A   the SI unit of temperature is the kelvin
B   infra-red thermography measures radiant heat
C   mercury thermometers have a rapid response time
D   mercury thermometers are influenced by atmospheric pressure
E   the Bourdon gauge can be adapted to measure temperature.

Paper VII   Answers

VII.1 FTTTT

A   Bicarbonate is formed by the action of the catalyst carbonic anhydrase.

D   The extracellular fluid volume is equivalent to about one-fifth body weight. Accounting for the intracellular bicarbonate brings this to about one-third body weight.

E   In potassium depletion, intracellular hydrogen ion concentration increases and bicarbonate is conserved as compensation.

VII.2 TTFTT

C   No reaction is 100% efficient. Aerobic oxidation is 60% efficient; the rest produces heat.

E   The respiratory quotient (RQ) is carbon dioxide production divided by oxygen uptake (at steady state). RQ for carbohydrates is lower than for fats (1.0 cf 0.7), and you can check this from a consideration of their molecular formulae.

VII.3 FFTFT

A   The intrinsic rhythm of the heart is altered by the autonomic nervous system.

B   *On average*, the output of the two ventricles must be the same; *beat-by-beat* there will be differences.

D   An increase in ventricular filling pressure *increases* stroke volume; this is Starling's law.

VII.4 TFFTT

B   Normal plasma phosphate is 0.8–1.4 mmol/l.

C   Serum phosphate concentrations are decreased by parathormone.

E   High energy nucleotides include adenosine triphosphate (ATP).

VII.5   FTFTF

The opioid peptide system is complicated. There are many different peptides, with precursors and pro-precursors, and they are found in the circulation, central nervous system and gastrointestinal tract. Do not try to commit too much detail to memory (details seem quite likely to change at frequent intervals).

AB   β-endorphin (itself cleaved from a larger molecule) contains 31 residues. The enkephalins are pentapeptides.

E   Substance P is a peptide, a *tachykinin*, but not an opioid peptide. The natural ligand for the μ-receptor is (at the time of writing) probably β-endorphin.

VII.6   TFTTT

B   It takes 2–3 days for the increase in circulating red cells.

C   The liver is the primary source of erythropoietin in the fetus and a secondary source in the adult.

D   Facilitation by catecholamines is β-adrenergic.

VII.7   TFFTF

A,B   In unmyelinated fibres, velocity is proportional to the square root of the diameter; in myelinated fibres, velocity is proportional directly to the diameter.

C   Altering ionic concentrations in a preparation in vitro affects threshold but not the velocity of an impulse once propagated. There is no effect in vivo.

E   Neurologists measure conduction velocities; and fast or slow pain is well recognised.

VII.8   TFTTF

A   Deficiency of glucocorticoids, of which cortisol is one, may cause water intoxication because a water load is excreted so slowly.

B,C   Cortisol increases sodium reabsorption and glomerular filtration. Overall, sodium excretion may increase.

D   Cortisol reduces the secretion of antidiuretic hormone.

E   Cortisol is diabetogenic, but increased glucose reabsorption is not the reason.

VII.9   TTTFF

A   Physiology is full of these figures – others are the effective area of the gastro-intestinal mucosa or the renal tubule. Don't try to memorise them, but they do occasionally crop up in MCQ examinations, and if you recognise a figure you will gain a mark. Otherwise leave it.

D,E   Answering true to either of these shows great ignorance of what happens in the lung.

VII.10   TFTFT

Exercise is a difficult topic for MCQs. Cardiorespiratory responses depend on time (what happens at the initiation of exercise is different to what happens in established exercise) and degree. The question here asks about 'moderate' exercise: what does that mean? The only useful answer we can give to that is to use your sense.

A   Decrease of diffusion distance is one of the adaptations that allow increased oxygen utilisation.

D   Arterial carbon dioxide tension is unchanged in moderate exercise.

E   The respiratory quotient increases as the oxygen debt is incurred.

VII.11   FTFFF

Penicillins affect bacterial cell wall synthesis.

A,D,E   Chloramphenicol, tetracyclines and the aminoglycosides inhibit protein synthesis within the cell at the bacterial ribosome.

C   An active metabolite of sulphonamides competes with para-amino benzoic acid, an essential compound of metabolism in bacteria.

VII.12   FTTFT

A   Hyoscine is a central depressant.

C   Hyoscine (and other similar drugs) are absorbed well from mucosal surfaces. Hyoscine is absorbed less well through the skin, but well enough to be useful when given as a skin patch for travel sickness.

D   The anticholinergic drugs are bronchodilators, the effect varying greatly with the cause of bronchodilation.

VII.13   TTTFF

D   Carbamazepine is chemically related to the tricyclic antidepressants but does not have anticholinergic side-effects.

E   The major tranquillisers are the drugs most likely to cause extrapyramidal symptoms.

VII.14   FTTFT

A   The effect of glyceryl trinitrate on myocardial oxygen consumption is indirect and quite complex.

D   Venous return is reduced by the venodilatation.

VII.15   FTFTF

A   Barbituric acid is malonyl urea: malonic acid and urea, not uric acid.

B   If the fat solubilities become too high they become toxic and convulsant.

C   Barbiturate anaesthesia was first used in the 1930s.

D   Methohexitone has some convulsant activity; compounds with double N-substitution even more.

E   Barbiturates *facilitate* GABA-ergic *inhibition*.

VII.16   FTTFF

A   It is a fluorinated methyl–ethyl ether.

B   What does 'very little' mean? It means: when we compare isoflurane with other similar drugs.

D   Its blood:gas solubility is 1.4; that of enflurane is 1.91.

E   Fluoride ion from methoxyflurane caused oliguric renal failure. Isoflurane does not.

VII.17   FTFFT

If the plasma concentration is high enough then any drug will cross the blood–brain barrier, but one must answer these questions sensibly.

A   Aminoglycosides are highly polar and little accumulates in the CNS. Remember, though, that they are ototoxic.

C   Penicillins will not cross readily when the meninges are normal.

D   Tubocurarine is highly polar.

VII.18   FTFTT

A   Streptokinase activates plasminogen and stimulates fibrinolysis.

C   Plasmin is activated to plasminogen, a proteinase.

VII.19 TFFTT

At the time of writing, desflurane is not yet available clinically in Britain, but candidates must know something about its properties.

A Desflurane's blood/gas partition coefficient is 0.42.
B Desflurane's MAC is about 6%, which is much higher than enflurane's.
C Desflurane's *low* boiling point and high vapour pressure (664 mmHg at 20°C) means special vaporisers are needed.

VII.20 TFTTT

There are many synthetic morphine-like drugs, and you cannot know details about them all. However, this question can be answered from a general knowledge of opioids and their receptors, and where nalbuphine fits into the scheme.

B Nalbuphine has a ceiling effect, but up to that dose (and therefore at equianalgesic doses) depresses ventilation equally.

VII.21 FFTTT

A,B Neostigmine's presynaptic effects increase the rate of repetitive firing after a single nerve impulse, though this is seen only in physiological preparations. Part of the reason that this phenomenon is not apparent clinically is that the predominant effect of neostigmine is on the muscarinic receptors, most importantly on the heart.

VII.22 TFFFF

A,B The light-emitting diodes use light in the red (660 nm) and infra-red (940 nm).
C All colour changes are sensed, but changes in the path length caused by arterial pulsation allow subtraction of changes caused by capillary and venous blood.
D At the isobestic point (800 nm), haemoglobin and oxyhaemoglobin have the same absorption, but pulse oximeters do not make use of this.
E In methaemoglobinaemia, pulse oximeters under-read at low saturations but over-read at high saturations.

VII.23 TTFTT

C,E Large tidal volumes lead to under-estimation of arterial partial pressures by diluting alveolar gas with atmospheric air; small tidal volumes do the same by risking dilution with dead space gas.
D The saturated vapour pressure of water is 6.3 kPa.

VII.24   TTFTF

A,B   This follows from the law of Mass Action, the dissociation constant of water, and the molecular weight of hydrogen (which is 1). Strictly, the temperature should be defined.

C   pH varies with the inverse of the carbon dioxide tension.

D   The activity is less than the concentration in concentrated solutions.

E   1 pH unit is a ten-fold change in hydrogen ion concentration.

VII.25   TTTFF

D   Doubling the radius of a tube increases laminar flow by 16 times.

E   Turbulent flow is proportional to the *square root*, not the square, of the pressure difference. Thus an equal pressure difference gives less flow if the flow is turbulent.

VII.26   TFFTF

'Normal' values vary somewhat between textbooks.

A   Sodium excretion is about 70–160 mmol per day.
B   Potassium excretion is about 40–120 mmol per day.
C   The normal adult does not excrete glucose in the urine.
D   Calcium excretion is about 2.5–7.5 mmol per day.
E   Creatinine excretion is about 12 mmol per day.

VII.27   TFFFF

B   24 V AC may not cause serious electrical shock but can cause microshock, which needs only very small currents.

C   The whole patient circuit is isolated from earth.

D   5% dextrose is a conductor, though not as good a conductor as saline.

E   Defibrillators contain batteries!

VII.28   FFTTT

A   Mains interference can be reduced by shielding the leads. Isolating from earth is a safety measure that has nothing to do with quality of the recorded signal.

B   Filters are usually put into circuits to *increase* the signal-to-noise ratio.

C   This is too complex to explain here.

VII.29   **TTFFT**

A,B,C   Work usually means mechanical work and is a form of energy, other forms being electrical energy and heat energy. Power is the rate of doing work.

D   Weight is a force. Force is mass multiplied by acceleration; the acceleration here is gravity, and at the surface of the earth mass and weight are equivalent.

E   No mechanical process is completely efficient; energy is wasted, for example, in frictional heat.

VII.30   **TTFFT**

C   Mercury thermometers take 2–3 min to reach equilibrium with their surroundings.

D   The mercury is enclosed in glass; atmospheric pressure can have no effect.

E   The Bourdon gauge is a pressure gauge; it can be filled with mercury and calibrated to read temperature directly.

Paper VIII Questions

VIII.1 **Some end-products of protein metabolism in man include:**
  A leucine
  B uric acid
  C urea
  D ammonia
  E sulphates.

VIII.2 **On rising from the supine to the upright position:**
  A the total peripheral resistance decreases
  B cerebral blood flow increases
  C the heart rate decreases
  D output of aldosterone and renin decreases
  E changes may be more marked if there is hypovolaemia.

VIII.3 **Which of the following are true of nervous transmission and innervation:**
  A myelin increases the electrical resistance of nerve fibres
  B most neurone to neurone transmission in mammals is electrical
  C 5-hydroxytryptamine is an inhibitory neuromuscular transmitter
  D gamma motoneurones innervate the muscle spindle
  E alpha motoneurones innervate voluntary muscle.

VIII.4 **The following hormones have their action via adenylate cyclase:**
  A parathyroid hormone
  B angiotensin
  C growth hormone
  D glucagon
  E β-adrenergic actions of catecholamines.

VIII.5 **The sodium pump:**
  A maintains the potential difference across cell membranes
  B involves activation of adenyl cyclase
  C exchanges three sodium ions for two potassium ions
  D is exclusive to excitable tissues
  E maintains an intracellular sodium concentration of 2–5 mmol/l.

VIII.6   In a consideration of human blood types:

    A   types A and B are Mendelian dominants
    B   the ABO group are classified by antigens in the membrane of red cells
    C   the ABO antigen system is exclusive to blood cells
    D   the most important reaction is of recipient plasma with donor cells
    E   'Rh-positive' means the individual will form anti-D agglutinin to D-positive cells.

VIII.7   Antidiuretic hormone:

    A   is a polypeptide
    B   production is sensitive to changes of osmolarity of 2–3 mosmol/l
    C   alters the permeability to water of the proximal convoluted tubule
    D   is controlled partly by activity in low-pressure stretch receptors
    E   is controlled partly by activity of osmoreceptors in the anterior hypothalamus.

VIII.8   ✓ Physiological dead space:

    A   includes the anatomical dead space
    B   is unchanged over a two-fold range of tidal volume
    C   accounts for the difference in composition between 'ideal' alveolar gas and mixed expired gas
    D   changes with posture
    E   is diffusion limited.

VIII.9   ✓ Hypocapnia:

    A   causes paraesthesiae
    B   causes dizziness
    C   causes vasoconstriction
    D   reduces secretion of cerebrospinal fluid
    E   decreases plasma sodium.

VIII.10   ✓ Intrapleural pressure:

    A   is subatmospheric in normal quiet breathing
    B   may reach -30 mmHg with increased inspiratory effort
    C   can be measured with an intragastric balloon
    D   is lower at the base than the apex when upright
    E   cannot rise above atmospheric pressure when the alveoli are open to the atmosphere.

VIII.11 **Propranolol:**
A   decreases coronary blood flow
B   worsens hay fever
C   is hypoglycaemic
D   blocks α-receptors in high dosage
E   has great inter-individual variability of oral absorption.

VIII.12 **In the treatment of paroxysmal ventricular tachycardia the following drugs may be used:**
A   digoxin
B   lignocaine
C   disopyramide
D   amiodarone
E   verapamil.

VIII.13 **When a drug is given:**
A   subcutaneously there is rapid initial absorption
B   intravenously the likelihood of serious anaphylaxis is lessened
C   sublingually there will not be first-pass metabolism in the liver
D   by aerosol absorption is almost instantaneous
E   there may be first-pass metabolism in the lung.

VIII.14 **Fat emulsions for parenteral nutrition (for example, Intralipid):**
A   can be given through a peripheral vein
B   must be stored in a refrigerator
C   must not have drugs added to the infusions
D   are isotonic
E   in 20% solution contain about 8000 kJ/l.

VIII.15 **Diethyl ether:**
A   causes profound peripheral vasodilatation
B   potentiates the action of non-depolarising muscle relaxants
C   is irritant to the upper respiratory tract
D   causes centrilobular hepatic necrosis
E   has an MAC of 1.9% in air.

VIII.16 **The binding of a drug to plasma proteins:**
A   prolongs its biological half-life
B   is likely to be different in arterial and venous blood
C   is only of importance to albumin
D   slows glomerular filtration of the drug
E   prevents renal tubular secretion of the drug.

VIII.17 Bronchodilation occurs with:

  A   isoflurane
  B   enflurane
  C   halothane
  D   diethyl ether
  E   nitrous oxide.

VIII.18 Propofol:

  A   is a substituted phenol
  B   has a total body clearance less than hepatic blood flow
  C   has no active metabolites
  D   has analgesic properties
  E   acts on central α_2-adrenoceptors.

VIII.19 Opioids:

  A   exert analgesic action via supraspinal μ receptors
  B   exert analgesic activity via spinal κ receptors
  C   exert respiratory depression primarily on central κ receptors
  D   are more likely to cause nausea if they act at μ receptors
  E   reduce lymphocyte activity in clinical dosage.

VIII.20 The following pairs of drugs have known interactions:

  A   rifampicin and phenytoin
  B   halothane and succinylcholine
  C   lithium and ketorolac
  D   phenobarbitone and penicillin
  E   vecuronium and cefuroxime.

VIII.21 When measuring the blood pressure indirectly:

  A   the width of the occluding cuff should be 20% greater than the diameter of the arm
  B   too narrow a cuff will give artificially high blood pressure
  C   the Korotkoff sounds have five phases
  D   the standard mercury column must be used vertically
  E   mercury columns should be calibrated regularly.

VIII.22 In the glucose tolerance test:

  A   intravenous glucose gives more reliable results than oral dosage
  B   subjects must be fasted
  C   diabetics have a slower rise in blood glucose
  D   the blood glucose of normal subjects returns to baseline in 90–120 min
  E   there is danger of hyperglycaemic coma.

VIII.23 **In the interpretation of statistics:**

    A a paired Student's t-test is more powerful than an unpaired t-test

    B 95% confidence limits correspond to a probability of 0.05

    C the standard error of the mean is the confidence limit of the mean

    D the F test compares variances

    E the sample means from a population will be normally distributed.

VIII.24 **The following are true of the intracellular fluid:**

    A it is approximately 40% of body weight

    B its volume can be measured directly with markers

    C inorganic phosphate is the most important anion

    D potassium concentration is approximately 150 mmol/l

    E its proportion varies little between tissues.

VIII.25 **In the movement of fluids and solutes:** *(Parbrook)*

    A diffusion is proportional to the permeability of the membrane

    B an impermeable anion will hinder diffusion of a permeable cation

    C the Gibbs–Donnan equilibrium depends upon the presence of non-diffusible ions

    D the osmotic pressure is that necessary to prevent diffusion of the solute

    E filtration depends on hydrostatic pressure.

VIII.26 **In gas liquid chromatography:**

    A there is partition of substances between a stationary phase and a moving phase

    B the column is packed with inert material

    C the carrier gas is often oxygen

    D substances are identified by their specific profiles at the detector

    E the technique is unsuitable for continuous measurement.

VIII.27 **For medical suction apparatus:** *(A h z)*

    A a larger reservoir will allow a greater suction pressure

    B a smaller reservoir will allow more rapid generation of suction pressure

    C the maximum suction pressure is about one-quarter of an atmosphere

    D rigid suction catheters have a side hole because of the Venturi effect

    E suction apparatus achieves a free flow of about 25 litres of air per minute.

VIII.28 Boyle's law:

    A concerns a fixed mass of gas

    B applies strictly only to ideal gases

    C states that, at constant temperature, volume varies directly with pressure

    D can be applied approximately to vapours

    E allows the calculation of the content of an oxygen cylinder.

VIII.29 When blood is taken for gas analysis:

    A the principle of oxygen tension measurement is polarography

    B total content of carbon dioxide is estimated from the pH

    C base excess is measured directly

    D venous blood does not need storage in ice

    E heparin of strength at least 25 000 IU/ml should be used.

VIII.30 For exponential processes:

    A the rate of change of a process is proportional to the size of the process at that time

    B passive exhalation is an exponential process

    C the theoretical total length of time taken by an exponential process is infinite

    D after five half-lives of exponential decay, the process will have fallen to 3% of its initial value

    E the time constant is the change in the process in one second.

Paper VIII Answers

VIII.1 **FFTFT**

A   Leucine is an amino acid, not an end-product.
B   Uric acid is a breakdown product of nucleotide bases not proteins.
D   In man, ammonia is converted to urea, mainly in the liver.
E   Sulphate ion comes from the sulphur-containing amino acids: cysteine and methionine.

VIII.2 **FFFFT**

The opposites of **A,B,C,D** are the normal responses to the decreased venous return, blood pressure, and other hydrostatic changes that occur on standing.

VIII.3 **TFFTT**

A   The myelin sheath is an insulating layer. Impulses travel faster in myelinated nerves not because of decreased resistance but because of saltatory conduction from node to node.
B   Electrical transmission between nerve cells occurs rarely if at all in mammals.
C   5-hydroxytryptamine (5-HT, or serotonin) is a transmitter in the lateral grey horns of the spinal cord, the brain stem and the hypothalamus
E   A very basic question.

VIII.4 **TFFTT**

C   The cellular action of growth hormone is at ribosomal level.

VIII.5 **TFTFF**

B   The enzyme for the sodium pump is a sodium-potassium-linked ATPase.
E   The normal intracellular sodium concentration is 5–10 mmol/l.

VIII.6   TTFTF
- **C**   The A and B antigens are found in many tissues.
- **E**   Rh-*negative* means the individual has no D antigen, and forms anti-D agglutinin when given D-positive cells.

VIII.7   TTFTT
- **C**   ADH acts on the distal convoluted tubule and collecting duct.

VIII.8   TFTTF
- **B**   Dead space increases with tidal volume, mainly because the large airways expand.
- **C**   'Ideal' alveolar gas is a theoretical concept. Dead space explains why it differs from mixed expired gas; shunt explains why its composition differs from that of arterial blood.
- **E**   Meaningless in this context: an example of 'diffusion limitation' would be the transfer of carbon monoxide in the lung.

VIII.9   TTTFT
- **D**   Intracerebral pressure is decreased, but because of decreased blood flow.
- **E**   Hypocapnia causes alkalosis, retention of hydrogen ions and consequent sodium loss.

VIII.10   TTFFF
You should be able to draw a graph of the intrathoracic pressures and volume over the respiratory cycle.
- **C**   An intragastric balloon measures intra-abdominal pressure. A lower oesophageal balloon will reflect intrapleural pressure.
- **D**   It is higher (i.e. less negative) for simple, gravitational, reasons.
- **E**   Forced expiration increases pressure above atmospheric. The alveoli (not the pleural cavity) are at atmospheric pressure when the airway is open to the atmosphere *and* there is no air flow.

VIII.11   FTTFT

A   Propranolol increases coronary flow by prolonging diastolic perfusion time.

D   Propranolol blocks β_1- and β_2-receptors, but not α-receptors.

E   There is a 20-fold range of plasma concentration after an oral dose.

VIII.12   FTTTF

The best treatment is cardioversion. Otherwise, lignocaine is a reasonable first choice. Disopyramide is also effective. Amiodarone must be given with care.

A   Digoxin is contraindicated.

E   Verapamil is not indicated; it is used in supraventricular tachycardias.

VIII.13   FFTTT

A   Subcutaneous absorption is variably slow, and sustained.

B   Anaphylaxis tends to be more severe if a drug is injected directly into the circulation.

C   Drainage from oral mucosa is to the superior vena cava.

VIII.14   TFTTT

AD   Intralipid can be given peripherally because it is isotonic.

B   Emulsions break down if frozen.

E   Each litre contains 8000 kJ/l from 200 g of fat emulsion, plus 11 g of glycerol to aid isotonicity.

VIII.15   FTTFT

Agents that are no longer available or rarely used should not appear in multiple choice examinations. However, ether is of such importance historically that it will always be relevant to ask questions about it.

A   Ether is a sympathetic stimulant, which is why it was such a safe agent.

B   It has an inhibitory action on descending pathways, as do all general anaesthetics, but also has an action at the neuromuscular junction.

D   Chloroform was hepatotoxic – directly so, unlike halothane.

VIII.16   TTFTF

B   Binding may be different because venous blood is more acid.

VIII.17   TTTTF

E   Nitrous oxide has no effect on the bronchial
        musculature.

VIII.18   TFTFF

A   Propofol is di-isopropyl phenol.
B   Total body clearance of propofol is greater than
        hepatic blood flow, which implies that other tissues are
        involved in its elimination.
E   There is evidence that central α_2-adrenoceptors are
        somehow involved in anaesthesia, but propofol does
        not act on them.

VIII.19   TTFTF

Our understanding of opioid receptors is far from complete.
C   Respiratory depression certainly involves μ receptors,
        and may involve others.
E   Altered white cell function has been described
        experimentally, but not clinically.

VIII.20   TFTFF

A   Rifampicin and phenytoin are both inducers of
        microsomal enzymes.
C   Ketorolac (in common with other NSAIDs) enhances
        proximal tubular reabsorption of sodium, and therefore
        of lithium.

VIII.21   TTTTF

E   Aneroid gauges should be calibrated. They are
        calibrated against mercury columns, which should be
        checked for blockages and leaks, but do not need
        calibrating.

VIII.22   FTFTF

A   The standard test is the oral glucose tolerance test.
C   Blood glucose rises more rapidly and to a higher peak
        in diabetics.

VIII.23   TTFTT

   C   The confidence limits of a mean can be calculated from the standard error of the mean.

VIII.24   TFTTF

   B   The volume is calculated by subtracting the extracellular fluid volume from the total body water.

   E   The proportion of intracellular fluid is less in fatty tissues.

VIII.25   TTTFT

   D   Osmotic pressure is that necessary to prevent diffusion of the *solvent*.

VIII.26   TTFFT

   C   The carrier gas is inert, and is commonly nitrogen.

   D   There are no specific profiles. You must know what you are looking for and compare prepared standards.

VIII.27   FTFFT

   A   Suction pressure is determined by the pump, not by the reservoir.

   C   Maximum suction pressure is about two-thirds of an atmosphere (0.67 bar).

   D   Suction catheters have a side hole to allow tissues sucked onto the end of the catheter to be released without having to turn off the apparatus.

VIII.28   TTFTT

B,D,E   The gas laws apply perfectly only to ideal gases, of which there are none but hydrogen is the closest. As an approximation, Boyle's law applies to all gases and vapours.

C   It is an inverse relation.

VIII.29   TFFFF

B   Total content of carbon dioxide is not used clinically (and could not be estimated from the pH anyway). Partial pressure is the most used measure.

C   Base excess is always a calculation.

D   Unless measurement is immediate, blood for gas analysis is stored on ice, whatever its source, to slow metabolism.

E   Heparin of 1000 IU/ml is sufficient; higher concentrations alter the pH.

VIII.30   TTTTF

D   After five half-lives, the quantity is reduced to $1/2^5 = 1/32 = 3.1\%$.

E   The time constant is the time at which the process would have been complete had the initial rate of change been maintained.

Paper IX   Questions

IX.1   **The following are true of the vesicles in the adrenal medulla:**

     A   they contain isoprenaline
     B   they contain catecholamines bound to the protein chromogranin
     C   they contain DOPA decarboxylase
     D   calcium ions are involved in the release process
     E   release of vesicles may be blocked by atropine.

IX.2   **The following are true of calcium:**

     A   the serum concentration is increased by parathormone
     B   approximately half the serum calcium is non-diffusible
     C   the non-diffusible serum fraction is mostly as relatively insoluble salts
     D   the tendency to tetany is proportional to the ratio of calcium to magnesium ions
     E   tetany arises because of overactivity of the neuromuscular junction.

IX.3   **The elastic tissue within the aortic wall:**

     A   prevents the aorta expanding with each beat
     B   maintains the onward flow of blood during ventricular diastole
     C   minimises the effects of changes in intrathoracic pressure upon aortic pressure
     D   converts the intermittent ejection from the heart to a continuous blood flow with minimal pressure loss
     E   maintains coronary perfusion pressure.

IX.4   **The following are true of magnesium:**

     A   it is the second most abundant intracellular cation
     B   approximately half the total body content is in bone
     C   it is important in neuromuscular activity
     D   growth hormone increases plasma magnesium
     E   it reduces peripheral vascular tone.

IX.5   **Aldosterone secretion:**

     A   is reduced during surgery
     B   is increased by inferior vena caval compression
     C   decreases on standing
     D   is reduced by low sodium intake
     E   is only secreted in conjunction with glucocorticoid release.

IX.6 **The normal blood clotting mechanism requires:**
- A activation of the kallikrein–kinin system
- B local vasoconstriction
- C fibrinolysis
- D phospholipids
- E factor XIII.

IX.7 **Nerve fibres:**
- A have a lower electrical resistance than surrounding body fluids and tissues
- B have velocities of propagation of impulses that are faster in larger fibres
- C have conduction velocities in muscle afferents of about 100 m/s
- D that are C pain fibres are unmyelinated
- E that are small are less susceptible to local anaesthetics.

IX.8 **In tubular reabsorption:**
- A seven-eighths of all reabsorption occurs within the proximal tubule
- B sodium reabsorption is mainly passive
- C the sodium pump is inhibited by ethacrynic acid
- D active proximal tubular reabsorption can be transport-maximum limited
- E glucuronides and sulphates are excreted mainly by filtration.

IX.9 **The inspired partial pressure of oxygen:**
- A is approximately 19.9 kPa (149 mmHg) in air saturated with water vapour at 37°C
- B can be increased by hyperventilation
- C is linearly related to the concentration of oxygen in the inspired air
- D is one of the terms in the alveolar air equation
- E is used to calculate ventilatory dead space.

IX.10 **The carriage of carbon dioxide by the blood:**
- A   is 85% as bicarbonate
- B   is partly as carboxyhaemoglobin
- C   influences the affinity of haemoglobin for oxygen
- D   is approximately 48 vol per cent in arterial blood
- E   is aided in exercise by selective ionisation of amphoteric proteins.

IX.11 **Haemoglobin in the normal adult:**
- A   is a tetramer
- B   is a molecule that changes shape during oxygenation
- C   98% of it is HbA
- D   may include some HbF in otherwise normal individuals
- E   has a molecular weight of about 65 000.

IX.12 **The following antibiotics may affect the fetus adversely :**
- A   streptomycin
- B   cloxacillin
- C   tetracycline
- D   tobramycin
- E   cefuroxime.

IX.13 **Ephedrine:**
- A   is both a direct and indirect acting sympathomimetic amine
- B   has both α and β effects
- C   is a monoamine-oxidase inhibitor
- D   induces bronchoconstriction
- E   reduces renal blood flow by causing local vasoconstriction.

IX.14 **Dobutamine:**
- A   has structural characteristics of both dopamine and isoprenaline
- B   is a synthetic sympathomimetic amine
- C   is a selective β_1-stimulant
- D   produces an increase in cardiac output without much increase in heart rate
- E   stimulates dopaminergic receptors in the kidney.

IX.15 **Metabolic acidosis inhibits the diuretic action of:**
- A   triamterene
- B   spironolactone
- C   frusemide
- D   chlorothiazide
- E   acetazolamide.

IX.16 Thiopentone:
A is formulated as the sodium salt to make it soluble in water
B has a high pH in solution
C acts in one arm–brain circulation time
D can be injected intra-arterially with care
E has a pK approximately the same as the normal pH of plasma.

IX.17 Nitrous oxide:
A forms a reversible complex with haemoglobin
B is 2% metabolised in the liver to nitric oxide
C induces diffusion hypoxia
D may worsen intestinal dilation
E interferes with vitamin B_{12} metabolism in the liver.

IX.18 Centrally acting anti-emetics include:
A metoclopramide
B ondansetron
C hyoscine
D cyclizine
E droperidol.

IX.19 Contraction of the pregnant uterus is stimulated by:
A progesterone
B vasopressin
C ergotamine
D histamine
E salbutamol.

IX.20 Dantrolene:
A acts by potentiating calcium release within the myocyte
B can be given orally for prophylaxis
C intravenous dosage is 300 mg/kg
D may cause muscle weakness
E depresses polysynaptic reflexes.

IX.21 Morphine:
A is a phenanthrene derivative
B is the analgesic of choice in biliary and renal colic
C has an anticholinergic effect
D decreases intracranial pressure
E is a good anticonvulsant.

IX.22 **The amount of gas dissolved in a liquid at constant ambient pressure at equilibrium depends on:**

- **A** the temperature of the liquid
- **B** the partial pressure of the gas
- **C** the diffusion coefficient
- **D** the solubility of the gas in the liquid
- **E** the critical temperature of the gas.

IX.23 **The normal partial pressure of:**

- **A** oxygen in the alveoli is 13.3 kPa (100 mmHg)
- **B** nitrogen in inspired air is 79.5 kPa (596 mmHg).
- **C** water vapour in the alveoli is 5.3 kPa (40 mmHg)
- **D** carbon dioxide in mixed expired gas is 4.3 kPa (32 mmHg)
- **E** oxygen in the right heart is 5.3 kPa (40 mmHg).

IX.24 **Linear regression analysis:**

- **A** applies a technique of minimising squared differences
- **B** can be used to analyse variables that are not distributed normally
- **C** yields a regression coefficient (the gradient)
- **D** yields an intercept that defines the position of the line
- **E** yields a correlation coefficient that is an indication of the 'goodness of fit' of the line to the data.

IX.25 **Colligative properties include or explain:**

- **A** the behaviour of azeotropes
- **B** the depression of freezing point of a solvent by a solute
- **C** the miscibility of different liquids
- **D** the Choanda effect
- **E** the effect of centrifugation on cell fractionation.

IX.26 **For electrical safety:**

- **A** there should be direct connection of an earth lead to the electrical chassis of patient monitoring systems to allow static charge to drain away
- **B** 'antistatic' operating theatre footwear has a low resistance to prevent charge building up
- **C** carbon-based materials are antistatic
- **D** endotracheal tubes are rendered conductive by the high humidity of gases passing through them
- **E** cotton possesses antistatic properties.

IX.27 **Concerning the Venturi principle:**
  A the potential energy of flowing gas is manifested as pressure
  B the kinetic energy of flowing gas is manifested as velocity
  C at the point of narrowing, flow and potential energy both increase
  D at the point of constriction, pressure increases
  E beyond the constriction, kinetic energy decreases and potential energy increases.

IX.28 **If a ventilator is a time-cycled flow generator:**
  A the tidal volume will decrease if the circuit resistance increases
  B the ventilatory frequency is a function of the tidal volume
  C increasing the ventilator minute volume increases the tidal volume and the inspiratory flow
  D increasing the flow decreases pulmonary compliance
  E tidal volume depends only upon ventilator settings.

IX.29 **An effective plenum anaesthetic vaporiser should include the following characteristics:**
  A high thermal capacity
  B back-flow restriction
  C active inbuilt temperature compensation
  D low resistance to gas flow
  E an increased output of anaesthetic vapour at low gas flows.

IX.30 **The following are true of humidity and humidifiers:**
  A less heat is lost from the body by breathing warm (30°C) dry gas than by breathing cool (15°C) moist gas
  B absolute humidity is constant at a given temperature and pressure
  C humidity can be measured with a Regnault's hygrometer
  D nebulised droplets should ideally be 20 μm in diameter
  E it is impossible to attain a relative humidity of more than 100%.

Paper IX   Answers

IX.1   FTFTF

A   Isoprenaline is a synthetic catecholamine.
C   This enzyme converts DOPA (dihydroxyphenylalanine) to dopamine, which then enters the granules. Dopamine is then converted to noradrenaline, the end-product in 15% of granules, or leaks out into the cytoplasm where monoamine oxidase converts it to adrenaline, which is the hormone in most of the vesicles.
E   Release is cholinergic, but is not blocked by atropine.

IX.2   TTFFF

C   The non-diffusible fraction of calcium is protein-bound not ionised: 75% to albumin, 25% to globulin.
D   The tendency to
tetany $= ([HCO_3^-][HPO_4^{2-}])/([Ca^{2+}][Mg^{2+}][H^+])$.
E   Tetany is caused by an increase in motor nerve activity that overrides depression of transmission at the neuromuscular junction.

IX.3   FTFFT

A   The aorta stretches during systole.
C   Effects of normal changes in intrathoracic pressure are insignificant.
D   Normal blood flow *is* intermittent, not continuous.
E   Myocardial perfusion occurs mostly during diastole.

IX.4   TTTFT

D   Growth hormone decreases serum magnesium by stimulating retention in bone and soft tissues.
E   Magnesium produces peripheral vasodilation and hypotension; it is used in some countries to treat severe pre-eclampsia.

IX.5   FTFFF

A   Aldosterone secretion is slightly *increased* during surgery.
C   Secretion *increases* secondary to secretion of renin in response to reduced blood pressure.
D   Secretion is increased to retain sodium.
E   Secreted alone when there is electrolyte imbalance.

IX.6   FTTTF

A   Kallikreins are formed from factor XII under the influence of plasmin and are responsible for the formation of bradykinin. This is a potent vasodilator involved in the inflammatory response but is not part of the clotting cascade.

B   Serotonin is the local vasoconstrictor.

C   Concurrent fibrinolysis prevents unlimited clotting in the blood stream.

D   Phospholipids are released from thrombocytes; they form complexes with the activated clotting factors.

E   Factor XIII is fibrin stabilising factor. It is not necessary in the initial stages of haemostasis.

IX.7   FTTTF

A   The simple electrical resistance of the membrane, like all membranes, is very high. It is the controlled changes in membrane permeabilities that enable nervous transmission.

B   In unmyelinated fibres, velocity is proportional to the square root of the diameter; in myelinated fibres, velocity is proportional directly to the diameter.

D   Aδ pain fibres are myelinated.

E   Smaller fibres are more susceptible to local anaesthetics.

IX.8   TFTTF

B   Sodium reabsorption is active mainly in the proximal tubule.

E   There is active transcellular excretion in the proximal convoluted tubule.

IX.9   TFTTF

A   (Ambient pressure – SVP of water) $\times F_IO_2$.

B   Hyperventilation increases the *alveolar* oxygen tension, but not the *inspired* oxygen tension.

C   This is Dalton's law of partial pressures.

D $P_AO_2 = P_IO_2 - P_ACO_2/R - F$; where P_IO_2 is calculated as in **A**, R is the respiratory quotient, and F is the nitrogen correction.

E   The Bohr equation for calculating dead space uses carbon dioxide not oxygen.

IX.10   TFTTF

A,D In 100 ml arterial blood about 42 ml carbon dioxide is transported as bicarbonate, 3 ml is dissolved and 3 ml is attached to haemoglobin. More carbon dioxide (up to 8 ml/dl) can be carried on reduced haemoglobin.

B Carboxyhaemoglobin is the complex formed with carbon monoxide. Read the question!

E This sounds very scientific and plausible but is nonsense. An amphoteric compound is one that can donate or accept a hydrogen ion. Proteins are amphoteric because they have both carboxyl and amino groups that can ionise, and this is one reason why they are effective buffers.

IX.11   TTTTT

A A tetramer is a molecule with four sub-units. Myoglobin is a monomer.

B The beta chains move relative to one another.

C The other 2% is HbA_2.

IX.12   TFTTF

A Streptomycin is ototoxic.

C Tetracycline may cause dental discoloration and is deposited in bones.

D Aminoglycosides are generally contraindicated in pregnancy because of the risk of renal and VIIIth nerve damage.

E There is no experimental evidence that the cephalosporins cause fetal damage, though they should only be given if really necessary.

IX.13   TTTFT

D Bronchodilation occurs because of the inhibition of bronchial smooth muscle.

E True: renal blood flow is not spared.

IX.14   TTTTF

C,D True: dobutamine is almost a pure inotrope. β_2 (+)

E Unlike dopamine, dobutamine does not produce specific renal vasodilatation; any improvement in urine flow occurs because of improved cardiac output.

IX.15   FFFTT

A Triamterene is a potassium-sparing diuretic, which seems to be better known by examiners than by prescribers, who are more likely to give the similar drug, amiloride.

B Spironolactone is an aldosterone antagonist.

IX.16 TTTFT

A   Six parts Na_2CO_3 to 100 parts thiopentone.
D   If injected intra-arterially it causes intense pain and spasm in the arterioles severe enough to cause death of the tissues supplied.

IX.17 FFTTT

A   Nitrous oxide does not combine with haemoglobin.
B   Nitric oxide is a toxic potential contaminant of commercial nitrous oxide; there is no significant metabolism of nitrous oxide.
D   Nitrous oxide diffuses down concentration gradients into any cavity containing air, such as bowel, middle ear or a pneumothorax.
E   A high concentration of nitrous oxide for over six hours inactivates the cobalamin component of methionine synthetase, leading to reduced synthesis of thymidine and DNA.

IX.18 TTTTT

A   Metoclopramide has both peripheral and central effects, acting by antagonism to dopaminergic receptors.
D   True: cyclizine is a competitive antihistamine whose main action is on the vomiting centre.
E   Droperidol acts centrally on dopaminergic receptors.

IX.19 FTTTF

A   Progesterone opposes the effect of oxytocin.
C   The drug in clinical use is *ergometrine*, but ergotamine is an oxytocic, though weaker than ergometrine.
E   Salbutamol is used to prevent premature labour.

IX.20 FTFTF

A   Exactly the opposite: dantrolene uncouples excitation-contraction coupling.
C   The intravenous dose is 1 mg/kg, repeated as necessary.
D   True: mechanical ventilation may be needed postoperatively.

IX.21 TFTFF

B   Morphine increases smooth muscle tone and may make it more difficult to pass the obstructing stone.
D   Morphine *increases* intracranial pressure probably directly, and certainly indirectly because of hypoventilation and carbon dioxide retention.
E   Morphine may produce excitation in some patients.

IX.22   TTFTF

A   The higher the temperature, the lower the solubility of a gas in a liquid.

B   This is from Henry's law.

C,E   Both irrelevant.

IX.23   TTTTT

D   Mixed expired gas is often forgotten – $P\bar{E}O_2$ 15.5 kPa (116 mmHg), $P\bar{E}CO_2$ 4.3 kPa (32 mmHg), $P\bar{E}H_2O$ 6.3 kPa (47 mmHg) and $P\bar{E}N_2$ 75 kPa (565 mmHg).

IX.24   TTTTT

B   Strictly, the variables should be normally distributed, or some non-parametric method should be used. In practice, one can apply the analysis to some non-normal data.

E   The correlation coefficient is usually denoted by r.

IX.25   TTFFF

Colligative properties are all related to osmolarity and include depression of freezing point, lowering of vapour pressure and raising of boiling point.

A   An azeotrope is a mixture of liquids whose boiling point remains constant during distillation. Ether/halothane azeotrope has been used clinically.

D   The Choanda effect is the boundary-layer effect used in the operation of devices relying on fluidic logic.

IX.26   FFTTT

A   Earth leads allow mains current to pass to earth if there is a fault in the monitor, but there should be no direct contact between the electrical chassis of the machine and the patient. Static electricity cannot be dissipated by this route.

B   No: they must have sufficient resistance to prevent the passage of current and danger of electrocution. However, they will offer little protection against mains electrocution.

IX.27 TTFFT

C   At the point of narrowing, potential energy decreases and kinetic energy increases.

D   At the point of constriction (which is just a different word for narrowing, but the examiners do not have a limited vocabulary), pressure decreases as velocity increases.

IX.28 FFTFT

A   Flow generators will maintain tidal volume as compliance changes until any safety blow-off valve in the patient system operates.

B   Tidal volume is the product of flow and inspiratory time, but the frequency is set by inspiratory and expiratory time.

D   Pulmonary compliance is independent of ventilator settings.

IX.29 TTFFF

A   High thermal capacity is necessary to prevent drops in temperature, and therefore output, at high gas flows.

B   Without back-flow restriction, output can become high with positive-pressure ventilation.

C   This is not essential, although nowadays usually incorporated. The 'Copper Kettle' vaporiser does not have inbuilt temperature compensation but is accurate.

D   Low internal resistance is necessary for draw-over, but not plenum, vaporisers.

E   Some vaporisers, such as the Fluotec 2, had this characteristic, but modern vaporisers do not.

IX.30 FFTFF

A   It takes little energy to alter the temperature of dry gases, but a considerable amount of heat is required to evaporate water to humidify dry gas.

B   False: absolute humidity depends upon the mass of water vapour present, which is obviously variable.

D   Drops 20 μm in diameter are deposited in the trachea or upper respiratory tract, which is a nuisance. Drops less than 1 μm in diameter are said to move in and out with airflow. These 'facts' are often quoted, but there is no direct evidence for them in human, or even animal, work.

E   A relative humidity of more than 100% is supersaturation, a clinical risk of efficient humidification.

Paper X Questions

X.1 The following are mitochondrial enzymes:

A cytochrome oxidase
B lactate dehydrogenase
C chymotrypsin
D succinate dehydrogenase
E arginase.

X.2 Physiological right-to-left shunt (venous admixture) is:

A partly flow from bronchial veins into pulmonary veins
B partly from Thebesian veins
C 20% of total pulmonary blood flow
D increased by pulmonary hypertension
E increased during sleep.

X.3 The following are true for stretch reflexes:

A they are a mechanism whereby stretch of a muscle results in contraction of the same muscle
B they cause increased tone in a stretched muscle
C in the decerebrate cat, transected below the superior colliculi, stretch reflexes are chiefly present in flexor muscles
D the knee-jerk is a monosynaptic stretch reflex
E they are 'all-or-none'.

X.4 The following are true of these hormones:

A thyroxine is a substituted amino acid
B prostaglandins are fatty acids
C steroids have their cellular effects via protein synthesis
D the peptide hormones are derived from β-lipotrophin
E corticosterone is the principal glucocorticoid in man.

X.5   Cell membranes:

A   are normally composed of a single lipid layer between two layers of protein

B   are crossed by lipid-soluble substances in proportion to the lipid-water partition coefficient

C   are penetrated by water-soluble substances proportionally to molecular size

D   are less permeable when the lipid solubility of a substance is decreased by ionisation

E   contain membrane transport proteins each specific for one substance, which are termed 'symports'.

X.6   Adverse drug reactions may be caused by:

A   idiosyncrasy

B   hypersensitivity

C   angioneurotic oedema

D   serum sickness

E   tachyphylaxis.

X.7   The clearance of a solute:

A   is the volume of plasma actually cleared of the solute

B   is measured in ml/min

C   is equal to the glomerular filtration rate

D   is greater if the solute is secreted by the tubules

E   is greater if the solute is osmotically active.

X.8   The following are true of sodium balance:

A   the major losses are by sweating

B   the kidney will have adjusted to a change in intake within 16 h

C   reabsorption of sodium is mainly in the distal convoluted tubule

D   about 22 000 mmol of sodium are filtered each day

E   in hyperaldosteronism there is increased total body sodium.

X.9   Carbon dioxide:

A   when at lower than normal tension produces cerebral vasodilatation

B   has a normal content in arterial blood of about 48 ml per 100 ml

C   affects the excitability of neurones in the reticular activating system

D   has a tension in mixed venous blood 0.8 kPa (6 mmHg) higher than in arterial blood

E   when bound to haemoglobin reduces the affinity of haemoglobin for oxygen.

X.10 The following statements about homeostasis are true:

A   the carotid and aortic bodies are sensitive to arterial blood pressure

B   hypotension produces increased baroreceptor discharge

C   increased plasma renin activity stimulates aldosterone production

D   posture influences aldosterone production

E   antidiuretic hormone secretion is affected by left atrial stretch receptors.

X.11 Pulmonary surfactant:

A   increases surface tension differentially in differently sized alveoli

B   helps prevent pulmonary oedema

C   increases alveolar ciliary motion

D   aids diffusion from the alveolus to the pulmonary capillary

E   is produced by the type II alveolar cells.

X.12 The following drugs may cause an increase in blood pressure:

A   phentolamine

B   guanethidine

C   glucagon

D   propranolol

E   terbutaline.

X.13 The following are positive inotropic agents:

A   labetalol

B   isoprenaline

C   protamine

D   prilocaine

E   calcium ions.

X.14   Epileptiform EEG activity may be induced by:

A   enflurane
B   midazolam
C   methohexitone
D   etomidate
E   isoflurane.

X.15   The following are true of sodium nitroprusside:

A   the intra-operative dose range is 0.5–6 mg/kg/min
B   metabolism to cyanide occurs non-enzymatically in blood
C   metabolism produces thiocyanate which is excreted in urine
D   it produces dilation predominantly of resistance vessels
E   administration is contraindicated in tobacco amblyopia.

X.16   Enflurane:

A   is an analgesic in sub-anaesthetic concentrations
B   has a MAC in man of 1.15% in air
C   is insoluble in rubber
D   will corrode metal components of vaporisers unless they are coated
E   potentiates the actions of non-depolarising muscle relaxants.

X.17   The absorption of weak acids from the stomach:

A   is at a rate directly proportional to the pH of gastric juice
B   is faster than that of weak bases
C   is by diffusion of the unionised acid across the gastric mucosa
D   is reduced in achlorhydria
E   does not occur during secretion of gastric acid induced by gastrin.

X.18   The following have anticonvulsant activity:

A   clonazepam
B   chlormethiazole
C   thiopentone
D   ketamine
E   chlorpromazine.

X.19   Heavy bupivacaine:

A   contains 0.5 mg/ml bupivacaine
B   has a specific gravity greater than that of cerebrospinal fluid
C   is presented as a 12% glucose solution
D   will be detectable in the mother's milk after use for caesarian section
E   will show accelerated onset of block if mixed with sodium bicarbonate.

X.20 Which of these statements about non-steroidal analgesics is true:

A paracetamol causes gastric erosions
B indomethacin is a conjugated salicylate
C aspirin lowers normal body temperature
D phenylbutazone may precipitate cardiac failure
E mefenamic acid may cause diarrhoea.

X.21 The following drugs should be avoided in patients with severe renal impairment (GFR < 10 ml/min):

A digoxin
B metformin
C gallamine
D disopyramide
E sulphadiazine.

X.22 The following are true of direct blood pressure measurement:

A it is always more accurate than indirect measurements
B the upper frequency response of suitable measuring apparatus should be 10 Hz
C the peak systolic pressure in the dorsalis pedis artery is often 10% higher than that in the aorta
D the resonant frequency of the system is increased by a shorter and stiffer catheter
E critical damping must be used if the system is to be accurate.

X.23 The following are true of ultrasound:

A low frequencies are audible to the human ear
B it is efficiently transmitted through air
C it is the Doppler shift of signals that allows visualisation of structures
D it has no adverse effects on human tissues
E it allows accurate measurement of the size of structures.

X.24 Errors in statistics:

A a Type I error is when the test predicts wrongly that an observation is from a different population

B a Type I error is the acceptance that some values that lie outside $p > 0.05$ may well be from that distribution

C a Type II error is when the test predicts wrongly that an observation is from the same population

D a Type II error is not finding a positive result when one actually exists

E Type II errors can be reduced by making trials double-blind.

X.25 In cardioversion:

A it is the voltage that is important

B only 10–30% of the energy applied to the chest wall will pass through the myocardium

C direct current capacitor discharge is the preferred technique

D if alternating current is used it must be synchronised with the R wave

E the maximum energy applied should not exceed 100 J.

X.26 The following are true statements about flow:

A at constant pressure, flow is directly proportional to resistance

B laminar flow is inversely proportional to viscosity

C doubling the radius of a tube reduces the resistance to flow to one-sixteenth

D in turbulent flow the velocity is greatest at the periphery of the column of fluid

E resistance to flow in a tube varies directly as the length.

X.27 If a liquid is allowed to vaporise in a mixture of gases to equilibrium, the partial pressure of the vapour in the mixture will depend on:

A the volume of the liquid

B the temperature of the liquid

C the surface area of the liquid

D atmospheric pressure

E the liquid density.

X.28 In the estimate of the arterial partial pressure of carbon dioxide:

A   the Fick principle can be used
B   the end-tidal partial pressure of carbon dioxide is a good estimate in fit healthy subjects
C   the end-tidal partial pressure of carbon dioxide is not a good estimate in infants
D   the rebreathing technique relies on equilibration between arterial and mixed venous carbon dioxide
E   Astrup interpolation depends on constructing buffer lines.

X.29 In devices for measuring temperature:

A   the electrical resistance of metal increases exponentially with temperature
B   the resistance of metal oxides used in thermistors decreases as temperature rises
C   the resistance change in a thermistor is linearly related to temperature
D   a thermocouple depends upon voltage change occurring in response to the temperature at the junction of two dissimilar metals
E   thermistors can be heat-sterilised routinely.

X.30 The following are true in the electrical handling of information:

A   a digital signal is one entered by typing at a keyboard
B   a digital signal provides a more accurate representation of a waveform than an analogue signal
C   signals must be converted to digital form before they can be stored
D   an input transducer converts a physiological signal to an electrical signal
E   computers can process both analogue and digital signals.

Paper X Answers

X.1 **TFFTF**

A Cytochrome oxidase is an enzyme in respiratory chain oxidation.

B Lactate dehydrogenase is a cytoplasmic enzyme that has five forms or isoenzymes. It catalyses the interconversion of pyruvate and lactate.

C Chymotrypsin is an exocrine pancreatic secretion.

D Succinate dehydrogenase is in the citric acid cycle.

E Arginase, in the urea cycle, catalyses the irreversible hydrolysis of arginine to yield urea and regenerate ornithine.

X.2 **TTFFT**

B Thebesian veins drain directly into the heart chambers.

C About 2% of total pulmonary blood flow.

D Shunt may well be increased in the conditions that give rise to pulmonary hypertension, but pulmonary hypertension does not, in itself, increase venous admixture.

X.3 **TFTTF**

B Tone is the contractile state of resting muscle and is mediated through the gamma efferents so that it is the same whatever the resting length of the muscle.

C True: local stimulation will cause flexion of the ipsilateral and extension of the contralateral side. This is one of the classic experiments in neurophysiology.

E Stretch reflexes are graded.

X.4 **TTTFF**

A Thyroxine is tetraiodothyronine.

D Not all peptide hormones are derived from β-lipotrophin.

E Cortisol is the main glucocorticoid, approximately seven times as much of it is secreted in 24 h than of corticosterone, and the plasma concentration is approximately 30 times greater.

X.5   FTTTF

A   Cell membranes are a *bilipid* layer sandwiched between protein.

E   A transport protein specific for one substance is a *uniport*; a *symport* protein requires the binding of more than one substance for transport to occur (for example, transport of glucose and sodium ions from the intestinal lumen to mucosal cells) , while an *antiport* exchanges one substance for another (for example, the Na^+/K^+ ATPase) .

X.6   TTFFF

C,D   Both these are symptoms, not causes.

E   Tachyphylaxis is not an adverse reaction, although sometimes it is an inconvenience.

X.7   FTFTF

A   Clearance is a theoretical value and is the volume of plasma that contains the same quantity of the solute as is present in the volume of urine that is formed in one minute.

C   Clearance is equal to glomerular filtration rate only if the substance is not secreted or absorbed by the tubules.

E   A red herring: osmotic properties of themselves do not affect clearance or excretion.

X.8   FFFTT

A   The major losses of sodium under normal circumstances are in the urine.

B   The kidney takes 3 days to adjust, though the process starts within hours.

C   Reabsorption is stimulated by aldosterone in the distal convoluted tubule but 90% of the reabsorption is in the proximal convoluted tubule and loop of Henle.

X.9   FTTTT

A   Hypocapnia causes vasoconstriction, which is why hyperventilation is used to reduce raised intracranial pressure.

B   Carbon dioxide is much more soluble than oxygen: blood contains more and at a lower partial pressure.

C   Neurones in the reticular activating system become progressively more excitable with an increasing carbon dioxide tension, until eventually carbon dioxide narcosis occurs.

D   This number is used in the rebreathing method of estimating the $PaCO_2$.

E   This is the Bohr effect.

X.10   FFTTT

A   The carotid and aortic bodies contain chemoreceptors; the baroreceptors are situated in the carotid sinus and aortic arch.

B   Hypertension increases baroreceptor discharge, which in turn inhibits tonic discharge of vasoconstrictor nerves and excites the cardio-inhibitory centre.

E   These are the body's main volume receptors; a reduction in circulating blood volume increases vasopressin release.

X.11   FTFFT

A   Surfactant *decreases* surface tension inversely with volume.

B   The high surface tension would otherwise be a force drawing water in to the alveoli.

D   Surfactant has no effect, of itself, on diffusion.

X.12   FTTFT

A   Phentolamine is an α-adrenergic blocker.

B   Guanethidine is a vasodilator. Although primarily hypotensive, intravenous injection causes hypertension at first because of release of transmitter from labile stores. Guanethidine used to be used in the treatment of *hyper*tension, but is now largely restricted to use in pain clinics for sympathetic limb pain.

C   Glucagon is an inotrope.

D   Propranolol is a β-blocker. Hypertension may occur on *withdrawal* of the drug, but it is contorted logic to claim that the propranolol has then *caused* the hypertension. Distorted logic is easy in the examination hall: take care!

E   Terbutaline is a β-agonist used as a bronchodilator and for the treatment of premature labour.

X.13   FTFFT

A   Labetalol (an α- and β-blocker) is a negative inotrope.

B   Isoprenaline is an almost pure β-agonist. Its most important effects are on heart rate, but it is also an inotrope and bronchodilator.

C   Protamine may cause bradycardia and hypotension, perhaps because of histamine release.

D   Most local anaesthetics depress the myocardium directly.

X.14   TFTFF

B   Midazolam, being a benzodiazepine, is a sedative.
D   Etomidate can be used as an anticonvulsant.
E   Unlike enflurane, isoflurane has not been associated with convulsions.

X.15   FTTFT

A   Dose range is 0.5–6 *micro*grams per kilogram per minute. Patients are put at risk regularly by doctors misreading or miswriting drug doses.
D   Sodium nitroprusside dilates all vessels.
E   There is an abnormality of cyanide metabolism in tobacco amblyopia.

X.16   FFFFT

A   Enflurane has little analgesic effect.
B   This is the MAC of isoflurane; the MAC of enflurane in air is 1.68.
C   Enflurane is readily soluble in rubber.
D   The combination of halothane and water vapour attacks brass, aluminium and lead; enflurane does not do this.

X.17   FTTTF

The higher the pH, the more ionised will be the weak acid, absorption will thus be less. Consideration of this will explain branches **A, D, C** and **D**.
E   Gastric acid is gastric acid no matter how its production is stimulated.

X.18   TTTFF

D,E   Careful, although they are not convulsant, they are not specifically anticonvulsants.

X.19   FTFTF

A   Heavy bupivacaine is a 0.5% solution and therefore contains 5 mg/ml bupivacaine.
B   The specific gravity of heavy bupivacaine is 1.026.
C   The glucose solution is 8%.
D   Bupivacaine does cross into breast milk, though the amount of systemic bupivacaine after spinal injection would be minute.
E   This technique speeds the onset of epidural anaesthesia, but the onset time of spinal bupivacaine is rapid enough.

X.20   FFFTT

- **B**   Indomethacin is an indole derivative, not a salicylate at all.
- **D**   Phenylbutazone causes fluid retention.
- **E**   Mefenamic acid (Ponstan®) is as powerful an analgesic as aspirin but not as powerful an anti-inflammatory drug.

X.21   FTTFT

All these drugs should be used with caution in patients with renal impairment but the question asks which should be *avoided* and quantifies the degree of impairment. According to the British National Formulary:

- **A**   Digoxin: up to 250 µg daily.
- **B**   Metformin: avoid because of the risk of lactic acidosis.
- **C**   Gallamine: avoid because of the risk of prolonged blockade. Gallamine is not much used now, but two facts about it often asked in MCQ papers are that it is excreted by the kidney, and that it has an anticholinergic action, which blocks the oculocardiac reflex.
- **D**   Disopyramide: reduce the dose.
- **E**   Sulphadiazine: avoid because of the high risk of tubular damage caused by crystalluria.

X.22   FFTFF

- **A**   Nonsense: the direct system may be incorrectly calibrated or the cannula may not be receiving a satisfactory signal.
- **B**   The upper frequency response for an accurately recorded pressure trace should be 30 Hz.
- **C**   Resonance occurs within the arterial tree as well as within the monitoring system.
- **E**   Critical damping is too severe for clinical use; the ideal is 70% of critical.

X.23   FFFFT

- **A**   Ultrasonic frequencies are, by definition, beyond the audible range; clinically used frequencies are MHz. The limit of audibility is around 20 kHz.
- **C**   Doppler shifts permit assessment of flow, but are not necessary to assess static structures.
- **D**   Powerful ultrasonic signals, for instance those in a lithotripter, may cause trauma.
- **E**   Hence using ultrasound to determine fetal size.

X.24   TTTTF

A,B   Different expressions of the same idea. Basically, a Type I error is a false positive.

C,D   Different expressions of the same idea. Basically, a Type II error is a false negative.

E   Blindness makes no difference. Factors such as sample size and the expected variability of the observations affect the likelihood of these errors.

X.25   FTTFF

A   It is the current that is important in cardioversion.

D   AC cannot be synchronised; the discharge is too long (0.1–0.2 s).

E   The maximum recommended energy is 300 J for an adult (though machines will usually discharge up to 400 J), 150 J for a child. Internal maximum is 80 J for an adult.

X.26   FTTFT

A   This *must* be incorrect because, whatever the type of flow and the exact relation of flow to resistance, flow must *decrease* as resistance increases.

B,C,E   These follow from the Hagen–Poiseuille formula. If a question of this type occurs, write down the appropriate formula *before* the exact wording of the question can confuse you. Anaesthetists are less familiar with this formula than they used to be.

D   Flow is always faster in the centre.

X.27   FTFFF

This is a restatement of the meaning of saturated vapour pressure: which depends only on the nature of the liquid and the temperature. With a small volume of liquid, you could argue that it would totally vaporise and not reach its SVP, in other words that **A** is true. This is not so: the question is of a state 'in equilibrium', which implies that some of the liquid remains as liquid.

X.28 **FTFFT**

A   Carbon dioxide can be used *as an indicator* for measuring blood flow *by* the Fick principle, but Fick is not used *to estimate* $PaCO_2$.

C   The higher metabolic rate and higher respiratory frequency will cause a less well-defined end-tidal plateau but the response time of the electrodes is fast enough to cope with this.

D   The equilibrium is between the bag and mixed venous blood. $PaCO_2$ is calculated on an assumption about the arterio-venous CO_2 difference: 0.8 kPa (6 mmHg).

X.29 **FTFTF**

A   Electrical resistance of metal increases linearly with temperature.

C   The resistance change in a thermistor is exponentially related to temperature.

E   Heat sterilisation alters the calibration of a thermistor.

X.30 **FFFTT**

A   A digital signal is nothing to do with digits meaning fingers; it means that the information is stored in numeric rather than physical form.

B   An analogue signal is a more accurate way of following a waveform, and all signals are generated initially in analogue form; but digital signals, once they have been derived, are unlikely to be distorted or degraded.

C   Information can be stored in many forms, including on smoke-drums (which is what physiologists used for many years), or gramophone records!

D   A transducer converts one form of energy to another; biological transducers almost always produce electrical outputs that can be interpreted by monitors.

E   Desktop computers are digital, but there are also analogue computers.

Paper XI Questions

XI.I **The following are transmitters at autonomic ganglia:**

A dobutamine
B acetyl choline
C gamma-amino butyric acid
D 5-hydroxytryptamine
E tyrosine.

XI.2 **For calcium:**

A active uptake is enhanced by vitamin D
B uptake is mainly in the proximal small bowel
C glucocorticoids decrease plasma ionised calcium
D its presence in bone is mainly as hydroxyapatite
E calcitonin is more important in regulation than parathyroid hormone.

XI.3 **Critical closing pressure of a blood vessel:**

A arises because of the elastic recoil in the vessel wall
B is more important in small vessels
C is generally greater than a pressure of zero
D is affected by activity of the precapillary sphincters
E is affected by the pressure of the surrounding tissues.

XI.4 **Bradykinin:**

A is a direct vasodilator
B increases capillary permeability
C stimulates the secretion of gastric acid
D causes pain when applied to a blister base
E is released from a precursor by kallikreins.

XI.5 **In the normal process of micturition:**

A control of the external sphincter is a learned ability
B the efferent limb of the voiding reflex is parasympathetic
C urine cannot be voided voluntarily until the bladder holds about 100 ml
D reflex contraction occurs at a bladder volume of 300–400 ml in the adult
E voluntary control of the flow of urine once initiated is via the pudendal nerves.

XI.6 **Platelets:**

A are the smallest nucleated circulating cells
B are activated by exposure to collagen
C contain ADP
D contain serotonin
E have their action partly by formation of thromboxane A_2.

XI.7   **The following are true for these sensory modalities:**
A   proprioception travels by the dorsal columns
B   temperature and pain travels by the contralateral
     spinothalamic tracts
C   fibres subserving fine touch cross before reaching the
     gracile and cuneate nuclei
D   there is no overlap for pain beyond two adjacent segments
E   referred pain travels by ganglionic autonomic-somatic
     collaterals.

XI.8   **In the excretion of water by healthy kidneys:**
A   about 180 litres of water are filtered daily
B   the excretion of solutes is not dependent on the volume of
     urine
C   as little as 0.3% of filtered water may be excreted
D   25% of water reabsorption occurs at the proximal
     convoluted tubule
E   15% of water reabsorption occurs at the loop of Henle.

XI.9   **In breathing:**
A   the diaphragm is the most important muscle
B   the external intercostal muscles are inspiratory muscles
C   paralysis of the diaphragm is not compatible with
     unsupported spontaneous ventilation
D   the work of quiet breathing is mostly to overcome airways
     resistance
E   the work of breathing is not a limiting factor in heavy
     exercise.

XI.10   **The oxyhaemoglobin dissociation curve is shifted to the
     right:**
A   if fetal haemoglobin is replaced by adult haemoglobin
B   by an increase in 2,3-diphosphoglycerate in the erythrocytes
C   by a raised temperature
D   by an increase in pH
E   by passage of blood through the lungs.

XI.11   **In humans atropine causes:**
A   secretion of anti-diuretic hormone
B   shortening of the PR interval on the electrocardiogram
C   relaxation of uterine muscle
D   relaxation of ureteric muscle
E   mydriasis.

XI.12 **Of calcium channel blockers:**

    A verapamil depresses conduction less than nifedipine
    B nifedipine is an effective vasodilator
    C diltiazem is not a myocardial depressant
    D nifedipine is effective rapidly sublingually / *intranasally*
    E their electrophysiological effects can be reversed by
       intravenous calcium.

XI.13 **Warfarin:**

    A is an antagonist of vitamin K
    B competes with phenylbutazone at plasma protein binding
       sites
    C does not affect already synthesised clotting factors
    D is contraindicated in severe hypertension
    E prevents normal fibrinolysis.

XI.14 **Metabolic alkalosis:**

    A is a result of treatment with frusemide
    B is a result of treatment with spironolactone
    C occurs after infusion but not ingestion of sodium
       bicarbonate
    D is a result of treatment with acetazolamide
    E can be treated with intravenous ammonium chloride.

XI.15 **Propofol:**

    A is a potent local histamine releaser
    B prevents the pressor response to laryngoscopy
    C depresses respiration in a dose-dependent fashion
    D has a beta half-life of about an hour
    E is insoluble in water.

XI.16 **Nitrous oxide:**

    A was first prepared by Joseph Priestley
    B does not affect cerebral blood flow
    C induces bone marrow depression following prolonged
       exposure
    D guarantees unconsciousness at 67% inspired if $PaCO_2$ is
       less than 20 mmHg
    E is 10 times more soluble in fat than in blood.

XI.17 **Inherited enzyme defects are clinically important when giving:**

    A non-steroidal anti-inflammatory drugs
    B succinylcholine
    C tetracycline
    D atracurium
    E thiopentone.

XI.18 Lignocaine:

    A is more than 95% metabolised by first pass effect if taken orally

    B is absorbed from the gastrointestinal tract

    C causes local vasodilatation

    D is absorbed from mucous membranes

    E is dealkylated in the liver.

XI.19 Dantrolene:

    A causes hepatic damage

    B aborts the symptoms of malignant hyperpyrexia in susceptible swine

    C produces severe myocardial depression

    D is only slightly soluble in water

    E hypersensitivity is a risk.

XI.20 Morphine:

    A crosses the placental barrier

    B relaxes the labouring uterus

    C relaxes the sphincter of Oddi

    D should be given with care to patients with myotonia

    E decreases plasma anti-diuretic hormone concentrations.

XI.21 Recombinant human erythropoietin:

    A can be taken orally

    B is effective in the anaemia of renal failure

    C is ineffective in subjects with normal erythropoiesis

    D may precipitate hypertension

    E causes allergic responses in about 5–20% of patients.

XI.22 When the concentration of a drug is plotted against the effect of the drug:

    A the plot is a straight line

    B the semi-logarithmic plot is a sigmoid curve

    C a non-competitive antagonist will reduce the slope

    D a rightwards shift of the plot indicates competitive antagonism

    E the reciprocal of the plot gives the clearance of the drug.

XI.23 Central venous pressure measurement:

    A is only an approximation unless the patient is supine

    B should be zeroed at the supra-sternal notch

    C gives normal values of right atrial pressure that should not exceed $+10\,cmH_2O$

    D is only an approximation unless the catheter is in the right atrium

    E can be measured accurately with an arterial pressure transducer.

XI.24 In the measurement of fluid volumes:

    A indocyanine green can be used to measure cardiac output

    B extracellular fluid volume is measured using radiolabelled water

    C intracellular fluid volume is measured indirectly from extracellular volume and total body water

    D plasma volume is measured with radio-iodinated serum albumin

    E chromium-labelled red cells are used to measure blood volume.

XI.25 Alveolar equilibration with a set inspired concentration of a volatile anaesthetic agent:

    A is more rapid if the cardiac output is high

    B is less rapid if the alveolar ventilation is low

    C is more rapid if MAC is low

    D is more rapid with a more volatile agent

    E is less rapid in children than in adults.

XI.26 Osmotic diuresis:

    A can be achieved with solutions of urea

    B may cause rebound cerebral oedema

    C ideally should be with a substance of low molecular weight

    D should be with a solute that is metabolised rapidly to limit the action

    E occurs with hyperglycaemia.

XI.27 The following are true for surgical diathermy:

    A the frequency is measured in MHz

    B it may inhibit the discharge of a pacemaker in fixed rate mode

    C more current flows through the tip of the diathermy forceps than through the plate

    D earthing prevents 'microshock'

    E the plate should not be placed over bony areas.

XI.28   The following are true of sterilisation:
  A   boiling for 15 min at 1 bar effectively guarantees sterility
  B   chemical sterilisation works by coagulation or alkylation of proteins
  C   sterilisation with ethylene oxide requires exposure for about 10 hours
  D   at least 4 h flushing with air is necessary to clear a ventilator after ethylene oxide sterilisation
  E   gamma irradiation is unsuitable for endotracheal tubes.

XI.29   Gas cylinders:

  A   are made of manganese steel
  B   have a coloured plastic ring at the neck to denote year of manufacture
  C   are tested every 2 years
  D   are available in sizes denoted by letters
  E   for operating theatres are covered with high resistance anti-static paint.

XI.30   The following are true of heat:
  A   specific heat capacity relates temperature increase to mass
  B   gases in general have high specific heat
  C   latent heat relates to the energy change on change of state
  D   one calorie is 4.18 joules
  E   heat is converted to energy when liquids vaporise.

Paper XI   Answers

XI.1   **FTFFF**
   A   Dopamine is a transmitter at ganglionic interneurones.
           Dobutamine is synthetic.
   C,D Gamma-amino butyric acid (GABA) and
           5-hydroxytryptamine are central neurotransmitters.
   E   Tyrosine is the amino acid from which the catecholamines
           are synthesised, but it is not a neurotransmitter.

XI.2   **TTTTF**
   C   Steroids lower plasma $[Ca^{2+}]$, and deplete the organic
           material of the bone matrix.
   E   The physiological role of calcitonin in humans is uncertain.

XI.3   **FTTTT**
   Critical closing pressure is the intraluminal pressure in a small
   vessel that is insufficient to maintain flow. The vessel then
   collapses even though the intraluminal pressure may not be
   zero. The importance of critical closing pressure is in capillary
   flow.

XI.4   **TTFTT**
   C   The kinins and histamine share a number of properties,
           but not release of gastric acid.

XI.5   **TTFTT**
   C   Urine can be voided voluntarily even when the bladder
           contains only a few millilitres.
   E   The external sphincter is supplied by the pudendal nerve
           (somatic efferents in segments S2–4).

XI.6   **FTTTT**
   A   Platelets are non-nucleated bodies.

XI.7   TTFFF

C   The pathway from fine touch decussates after the nuclei.
D   The abolition of pain would be far easier if this were true.
E   Referred pain is a poorly understood and complex process. Integration probably takes place higher in the nervous system than the ganglia. 'Ganglionic autonomic–somatic collaterals' is a fine-sounding phrase, but the answer is 'false'.

XI.8   TTTFT

A,C   You may not know the figures for the daily filtered water load and percentage minimal urine excretion, but you should be able to calculate them.
B   The excretion of solutes is limited by the volume of urine if there is renal insufficiency.
D   70% of water reabsorption occurs at the proximal convoluted tubule.

XI.9   TTFFT

C   A patient with a paralysed diaphragm can just maintain sufficient ventilation.
D   The work of quiet breathing is mostly overcoming elastic recoil.
E   Heavy exercise is limited by supply of oxygen to the mitochondria; the work of breathing (less than 3% of the total output) can be ignored.

XI.10   TTTFF

Draw the curve first.
A   Adult haemoglobin has a lower affinity.
E   Passage through the lungs decreases the carbon dioxide tension and increases the pH: the curve shifts to the left.

XI.11   FTFTT

C   Uterine muscle has parasympathetic innervation, but the effect of atropine (and similar drugs) in humans is negligible.
E   Mydriasis is dilatation of the pupils.

XI.12   FTTTF

A   Verapamil has a more depressant action on conduction than nifedipine or diltiazem.

E   Intravenous calcium can reverse the haemodynamic effects, but not the electrophysiological ones.

XI.13   TTTTF

C   The action of warfarin is to prevent (via its effect on vitamin K) carboxylation of newly synthesised factors.

E   Warfarin does not interfere with the fibrinolytic cascade.

XI.14   TFFFT

A,B   The mode of action of diuretics is quite complicated but often asked: look it up.

C   If an alkali is soluble (which sodium bicarbonate is) it will be absorbed.

D   Acetazolamide (a carbonic anhydrase inhibitor) can be used to treat metabolic alkalosis.

XI.15   FFTTT

A   Propofol does not cause release of histamine. It can cause pain on injection, but the reason is unknown.

D   Values for pharmacokinetic parameters can vary widely between studies, but 60 min for the β half-life is a fair average. Do not waste time trying to learn these values for all the agents you use. You should know roughly how intravenous agents compare with one another.

E   Propofol is solubilised as an emulsion.

XI.16   TTTFF   → ↑ ICP, ↑ br. flow [A-2]

D   MAC is affected by $PaCO_2$, but not that much.

E   The oil/water partition coefficient of nitrous oxide is 3.2.

XI.17   FTFFT

A   We are not aware of any defects with which NSAIDs cause problems.

B   Pseudocholinesterase deficiency.

D   Atracurium is partly metabolised by pseudocholinesterase, but Hofmann degradation is more important.

E   Porphyria is an enzyme defect.

XI.18   FTTTT

A   Lignocaine is well absorbed but two-thirds is removed by first pass elimination and hence plasma concentrations are low and unpredictable.

XI.19   TTFTF

A   Hepatotoxicity is a problem of long-term use (the drug is used in spasticity).

B   The Part 2 examination is in human physiology and pharmacology, but much of that is based on animal work. The pig model is still important in malignant hyperpyrexia.

C   Dantrolene is only a mild myocardial depressant.

D   Dantrolene is much more soluble in alkaline solution.

E   Hypersensitivity has not been demonstrated.

XI.20   TFFTF

B   Morphine has no effect on the uterus.

C   Morphine causes sphincteric spasm, not relieved by atropine.

E   Morphine increases plasma concentrations of anti-diuretic hormone directly. Postoperatively, effective pain relief will reduce abnormally increased concentrations (an indirect effect of morphine).

XI.21   FTFTF

A   Recombinant human erythropoietin, often referred to as epo, is injected intravenously or subcutaneously.

D   Hypertension may occur if the haematocrit is allowed to increase too rapidly.

E   Allergic reactions have not been reported.

XI.22   FTTTF

A,B   The plot is a hyperbola, of which the semi-logarithmic plot (log dose against effect) is a sigmoid.

C,D   What antagonists do to dose-effect curves can be complicated; these are the 'classical' results.

E   Clearance is pharmacokinetics; dose-effect is pharmacodynamics.

XI.23   FFTFT

A,B   The posture does not matter. The supra-sternal notch is a convenient zero but is above the right atrium when supine. It doesn't matter where zero is if it is kept constant and allowance is made for the vertical distance from the atrium.

D   The catheter does not even have to be in the chest at all; the requirement is for a continuous column of fluid between catheter tip and right atrium.

E   Transducers are not specific for a particular measurement, but will need recalibrating for lower pressures.

XI.24   TFTTT

A   The use of indocyanine green has been largely replaced by thermodilution.

B   Water is freely diffusible, so labelled water cannot define one compartment.

E   Labelled red cells allow estimation of blood volume, provided the haematocrit is known.

XI.25   FTFFT

If you marked **A** and **B** incorrectly you lack the basic ideas of the uptake of volatile agents. Go to the standard textbooks, and ask for tutorial help.

C   The question asks about speed of equilibration, not speed of induction.

D   There is no relation between volatility and rate of induction.

E   Cardiac output is relatively higher than minute ventilation in children.

XI.26   TTTFT

B   The solute (usually mannitol) enters brain cells and 'holds' the water after the systemic loss of fluid through the kidneys.

D   Osmotic diuretics depend on not being metabolised.

XI.27   TFFFT

B   A pacemaker in *demand* mode may 'see' the diathermy as an R wave and fail to pace.

C   The total current flowing in an electrical circuit is constant; this will be true for diathermy unless a fault develops allowing parallel current flow to earth.

D   A complex subject. Patients are safer if the device is isolated from earth.

E   Bone has high resistance.

XI.28 FTTTF

A   Boiling at 1 bar (that is, at 100°C) does not guarantee killing all bacterial spores.

C,D You should know that ventilators can be sterilised with ethylene oxide (though it may be more Part 3 information than Part 2). Remembering the times is more difficult, but we ask the question to remind you that you cannot know everything.

E   Gamma irradiation is the usual method of sterilisation during manufacture.

XI.29 TFFTF   *Molybdenum Steel*

B   The coloured discs denote the year in which the cylinder was last tested.

C   The interval between cylinder testing is 5–10 years.

XI.30 TFTTF

B   Gases have low specific heat. Water has a high specific heat.

E   Heat *is* a form of energy.

Paper XII   Questions

XII.1   In intermediary metabolism:

A   the interconversion of lactate and pyruvate is catalysed by
     lactate dehydrogenase
B   the citric acid cycle produces pyruvate
C   ketone bodies are metabolised preferentially in the liver
D   ketone bodies form in starvation
E   fatty acids are synthesised from acetyl-CoA.

XII.2   In the myocardium:

A   cells have an internal resting potential of $+90$ mV
B   the plateau potential is due to calcium channels
C   metabolism is predominantly aerobic
D   there is no myoglobin
E   cells contain myosin but not actin.

XII.3   The stretch reflex (for example, the knee jerk):

A   cannot be elicited if the motor cortex is not intact
B   is an example of an axon reflex
C   is brisker in long motor tract damage
D   is brisker ipsilaterally below the lesion in hemisection of the
     spinal cord
E   is inhibited by activity from Golgi tendon organs.

XII.4   Growth hormone:

A   increases output of glucose from the liver
B   increases intestinal calcium absorption
C   decreases utilisation of fatty acids
D   production is decreased by hypothalamic somatostatin
E   exerts some of its effects via somatomedins.

XII.5   Gastric acid:

A   is isotonic
B   secretion is stimulated by hypoglycaemia
C   is secreted by the parietal cells
D   secretion is abolished by vagotomy
E   secretion is inhibited by gastric distension.

XII.6   The following are true of immunoglobulins:

A   IgG has higher concentrations in the plasma than other immunoglobulins

B   IgM causes complement fixation

C   IgA is present in seromucous secretions

D   atopic individuals are identified by high concentrations of reaginic antibody

E   the antibody responsible for thiopentone hypersensitivity is probably an IgE.

XII.7   In the liver:

A   oxygenated blood is delivered by branches of the hepatic artery

B   total blood flow is half the cardiac output

C   flow is from the periphery of the acini to the hepatic vein at the centre

D   portal venous pressure is about 10 mmHg

E   adenosine is important in local regulation of blood flow.

XII.8   At reduced body temperature:

A   oxygen and carbon dioxide are less soluble in body fluids

B   the oxyhaemoglobin dissociation curve shifts to the left

C   carbon dioxide carrying capacity of the blood is increased

D   oxygen requirements at 30°C are about 70% of normal

E   blood viscosity is decreased.

XII.9   Recognised non-respiratory functions of the lung include:

A   activation of angiotensin I

B   metabolism of circulating adenine nucleotides

C   the synthesis of circulating kallikrein

D   the inactivation of circulating bradykinin

E   the inactivation of circulating adrenaline.

XII.10   When considering compliance of the lungs:

A   dynamic compliance can be measured only during mechanical ventilation

B   compliance is at its lowest over the normal tidal range

C   compliance is increased at high lung volume

D   dynamic compliance is the same as chest wall compliance in a fit young adult

E   the normal value is about $200 \, ml/cmH_2O$.

XII.11 Levodopa:

  A is a precursor of dopamine
  B is actively transported across the blood-brain barrier
  C may precipitate malignant neuroleptic syndrome on sudden withdrawal
  D commonly causes postural hypotension when therapy is first started
  E increases the dose needed for intravenous induction of anaesthesia.

XII.12 Clonidine:

  A is a partial agonist at α_2-adrenoceptors
  B can cause hypertension if infused intravenously
  C is well absorbed when taken orally
  D anxiety is an important side-effect
  E reduces cardiac contractility.

XII.13 Intracranial pressure is increased by:

  A halothane
  B suxamethonium
  C morphine
  D nitroglycerine
  E etomidate.

XII.14 Monoamine oxidase inhibitors include:

  A tranylcypromine
  B phenelzine
  C dothiepin
  D isocarboxazid
  E fluphenazine.

XII.15 Sevoflurane:

  A has an MAC of 2%
  B cannot be administered from a conventional vaporiser
  C is metabolised with the formation of free fluoride ions
  D is broken down by soda lime
  E is a respiratory depressant.

XII.16 Evidence for the existence of drug receptors includes the following:

    A some drugs act at great dilution

    B access to the site of action is faster than could be explained by diffusion alone

    C concentration of drugs occurs at special regions of cell membranes

    D active drugs have a specific stereochemistry

    E a plot of dose against response is not linear.

XII.17 Hartmann's solution contains:

    A 141 mmol sodium

    B 101 mmol chloride

    C 5 mmol potassium

    D 29 mmol bicarbonate

    E 2 mmol calcium.

XII.18 Local anaesthetics such as lignocaine and bupivacaine:

    A prevent sodium conduction in nerve fibres

    B bind at the same site as tetrodotoxin

    C block sensory fibres preferentially

    D block smaller fibres before larger fibres

    E affect tetanised nerve more rapidly than resting nerve.

XII.19 The following statements are true of these non-narcotic analgesics:

    A aspirin is absorbed best in the ionised form

    B indomethacin can cause bleeding from any point in the gastrointestinal tract

    C diclofenac may cause renal damage

    D soluble aspirin tablets form calcium acetylsalicylate in water

    E phenacetin is addictive.

XII.20 Omeprazole:

    A acts by inhibiting the sodium ATPase pump

    B does not affect renal tubular acidification

    C is useful for reducing gastric volume

    D has an action that usefully outlasts its administration

    E must be given with careful monitoring of hepatic function.

XII.21 Aminophylline:
A   is a methylxanthine
B   interacts with adenosine receptors
C   is a central respiratory depressant
D   increases cardiac contractility
E   causes generalised epileptiform seizures.

XII.22 Automated oscillometric measurement of blood pressure (e.g. Dinamap®):
A   usually works from a double cuff
B   at normal systolic pressures is accurate to within 5 mmHg of simultaneous intra-arterial values
C   is more accurate if repeated at one-minute intervals
D   gives mean pressure as the pressure at greatest oscillation
E   is microprocessor controlled.

XII.23 A ventilatory flow-volume loop:
A   usually has volume on the x-axis (horizontal axis)
B   gives an enclosed area that is inversely related to time
C   is used in the assessment of airways resistance
D   is used in the assessment of airways compliance
E   is used in the measurement of closing volume.

XII.24 In statistics:
A   a Normal (Gaussian) distribution has 68% of observations lying within one standard error of the mean
B   Student's 't' test is so called because it is for beginners in statistics
C   the chi squared test is used to compare frequencies
D   if $p < 0.001$ there is no possibility that it could have occurred by chance
E   the sum of observations divided by the number of observations is the median value.

XII.25   The following are true statements about pH and ionic dissociation:

A   a weak base will be 1000 times less ionised at a pH of 7 than at pH of 4

B   a drug with a high pK will be a base

C   the pH is inversely proportional to the hydrogen ion concentration

D   a pH of 7.1 corresponds to a hydrogen ion concentration of 80 nmol/l

E   a compound can have more than one pK.

XII.26   At the time of the peak of the normal R wave of the electrocardiogram:

A   aortic pressure is about 80 mmHg

B   left ventricular pressure is at its lowest

C   the v wave occurs in the jugular venous pulse

D   left ventricular volume is at its highest

E   pulmonary artery wedge pressure most accurately reflects left atrial pressure.

XII.27   Plenum vaporisers:

A   are not suitable for use with anaesthetic techniques using spontaneous ventilation

B   generally rely on full saturation of gas entering the vaporising chamber

C   have a performance generally independent of fresh gas flow

D   cannot be used 'in circuit'

E   at a given setting, deliver the same partial pressure of vapour at 2 bar.

XII.28   The following are true of the behaviour of gases:

A   Boyle's law relates pressure and volume

B   Charles's law relates volume and temperature

C   the universal gas law includes a term for mass

D   the partial pressure of a gas in a mixture is not affected by the other gases in the mixture

E   an adiabatic change is one in which temperature is held constant.

XII.29   These are true in the SI system of measurement:

A   the basic unit of mass is the kilogram

B   pico is the prefix denoting 10^{-12}

C   the Hertz is the derived unit of frequency

D   it is allowable to use temperature on the centigrade (Celsius) scale

E   the units of resistance to fluid flow are $kg.m^{-4}.s^{-3}$.

XII.30 Isotopes of an element:

    A have the same number of protons

    B have different numbers of neutrons

    C are chemically identical

    D have the same mass number

    E cannot be separated physically.

Paper XII Answers

XII.1 **TFFTT**

 A LDH catalyses the interconversion of lactate and pyruvate, the co-enzyme (NAD: nicotinamide adenine dinucleotide) accepting the hydrogen from lactate.
 B Pyruvate enters the citric acid cycle non-reversibly.
 C The liver synthesises ketone bodies, but metabolises them poorly.
 E Acetyl-CoA is an important intermediate metabolite.

XII.2 **FTTFF**

 A Correct figure, but cells are negative inside: – 90 mV.
 D The myocardium has a high content of myoglobin.
 E The contractile proteins in heart muscle are the same as in skeletal muscle.

XII.3 **FFTTF**

 A The stretch reflex is affected by higher centres, but not dependent on them.
 B The stretch reflex is a monosynaptic reflex; an axon reflex does not require a synapse.
 E Activity from Golgi tendon organ feedback is by Ib afferents.

XII.4 **TTFTT**

 C Growth hormone is important in the release of energy from free fatty acids, though the process takes some hours. Free fatty acids are a source of energy in hypoglycaemia, fasting and stress.
 E Effects on growth and protein metabolism are via somatomedins, but not effects on carbohydrate metabolism. Somatomedins are chemically related to insulin.

XII.5 **TTTFF**

 A,C Pure parietal cell secretion is probably isotonic hydrochloric acid. The pH will be less than 1.
 D Vagotomy will not abolish secretion regulated by local influences.
 E Secretion is stimulated by gastric distension.

XII.6   TTTFT

D,E   Atopic individuals do not always have high concentrations of reaginic antibody (IgE). Concentrations are likely to be high when an individual is chronically exposed to an antigen to which they are sensitive, for example during the hay fever season.

XII.7   TFFTT

B   Resting hepatic blood flow is about 30% of cardiac output. The question does not specify resting, but questions that do not specify conditions should be assumed to refer to the normal adult under normal conditions at rest.

C   Flow is in the opposite direction: from the terminal branches of the portal vein and hepatic artery in the centre, to the terminal hepatic venules at the periphery.

E   Adenosine vasodilates the terminal arterioles; when flow increases the adenosine is washed away.

XII.8   FTTTF

A,B,C   Gases in general are more soluble in liquids at lower temperatures. As a separate phenomenon the affinity of haemoglobin for oxygen is increased.

E   Blood viscosity is increased in hypothermia.

XII.9   TTTTF

A,C,D   The metabolic function of the lung is complicated: the converting enzyme responsible for activating angiotensin I to the active angiotensin II also inactivates bradykinin; but the lung also synthesises kallikrein, which produces bradykinin from its precursor.

XII.10   FFFFT

Compliance is the ease with which the thorax distends to a pressure change ('volume per pressure'). It must therefore be greater when the lungs are less full (**B,C**) provided that the airways have not collapsed. Compliance can be measured either as static or dynamic compliance, breathing spontaneously or with mechanical ventilation (**A**).

D   Compliance is a function of both lung and chest wall compliance.

XII.11   TTTTF

A,B   Levodopa is used in Parkinsonism. Dopamine itself has no effect because it is decarboxylated in the periphery.

D   The mechanism for hypotension is unclear.

E   There is no evidence that levodopa has any effect on induction doses.

XII.12   TTTFF

A,B   Clonidine has different actions if given acutely or chronically. It is certainly a partial α-agonist but its most important anti-hypertensive action is probably via central receptors.

D   Sedation is an important side-effect. The relation between central adrenoceptors and anaesthesia is currently under investigation.

E   Cardiac output is decreased, but contractility is unaffected.

XII.13   TTFTF

A   The increase is slight unless concentrations of halothane are high, or carbon dioxide is allowed to accumulate.

B   Suxamethonium causes a small, transient, rise, which is clinically unimportant.

C   Intracranial pressure is not increased by opioids if $PaCO_2$ is normal.

D   Vasodilators increase intracranial pressure.

E   Etomidate sedation reduces raised intracranial pressure.

XII.14   TTFTF

Monoamine oxidase inhibitors may be coming back into fashion.

C   Dothiepin is a tricyclic antidepressant.

E   Fluphenazine is a phenothiazine used in the treatment of schizophrenia and related psychoses.

XII.15   TFTTT

At the time of writing, sevoflurane is not commercially available in the UK.

B   Desflurane (also not yet available) has to be delivered from a heated, pressurised vaporiser.

C   Release of free fluoride is about the same as from enflurane, though toxicity has not been reported.

XII.16   TFTTF

One of the major topics of general pharmacology and one that you should read about in some detail.

B   Ease of passing membranes has nothing to do with subsequent mode of action.

E   Many pharmacological and physiological responses are logarithmic; this does not imply receptors.

XII.17   FFTFT

You must know the composition of fluids that you use every day. Hartmann's contains 131 mmol sodium, 111 mmol chloride, 29 mmol lactate (which is metabolised to bicarbonate).

XII.18   TFFTT

B   Local anaesthetics and tetrodotoxin bind at opposite ends of the sodium channel.

C,D   In general (though it is complicated) smaller fibres are more susceptible than larger; there is no selectivity for sensory fibres.

E   Tetanised nerve is blocked more rapidly, perhaps because the sodium channels are in the open state more of the time.

XII.19   FTTTF

A   Drugs are usually best absorbed in the un-ionised, lipid-soluble, form.

C   It is becoming increasingly recognised that NSAIDs worsen already impaired renal function.

D   Soluble aspirin tablets are aspirin, citric acid and calcium carbonate.

E   The story of phenacetin 'addiction' in a town in Sweden is interesting, but phenacetin is not pharmacologically addictive.

XII.20   FTFTF

A   Omeprazole inhibits the hydrogen ion-potassium ATPase, the so-called proton pump.

C   Omeprazole has little affect on gastric volume.

D   Its action persists after it can no longer be measured in the plasma.

E   There may be slight alterations in plasma aminotransferases, but not enough to warrant monitoring.

XII.21   TTFTT

Methylxanthines are an almost traditional treatment for asthma. They have many effects, and their mode of action for these many effects are far from clear. You should be aware that some regard aminophylline as a completely outdated drug.

C   Aminophylline (in common with other methylxanthines such as theophylline and caffeine) is a central stimulant, and stimulates the respiratory centre.

XII.22   FFFTT

A   Most automatic oscillometric devices have a single cuff.

B   The 95% confidence limits of a single reading of 120 mmHg are ± 18 mmHg.

C   Repeated measurement may give a better idea of what the true pressure is (although one-minute intervals is risking inaccuracy because of venous engorgement) but the readings do not become any more accurate.

XII.23   TTTFF

A,B   Volume is plotted horizontally and flow vertically. Greater flow for a given volume gives a greater vertical measure – that volume being moved in a shorter time.

C,D   Airways resistance affects flow; compliance (volume per pressure change) has no units of time.

E   Closing volume is measured as concentration of marker gas against expired volume.

XII.24   FFTFF

A   68% of observations lie within one standard deviation of the mean.

B   The 't' test is named after the man who described the distribution. He published the work under the pseudonym 'Student'.

D   If you answered true then you have a poor understanding of the rudiments of statistics and should seek help. There is always a possibility of a chance occurrence; if $p < 0.001$ that chance is less than one in 1000.

E   Sum divided by number is the mean; the median is the middlemost value (the same as the mean for a normal distribution).

XII.25   TFFTT

An understanding of logarithms and pH units will explain these answers but a full consideration is outside the scope of this book.

A   Three pH units = 1000 times.
B   The pK does not define the drug. A high pK means a strong base or a weak acid.
C   pH is inversely *related* to the hydrogen ion concentration, but the relation is logarithmic, not simple proportionality.
E   Any compound with more than one ionisable group (for example, amphoteric proteins) will have a pK for each group, which will not necessarily be the same.

XII.26   TFFTF

Questions on the timing of events in the cardiac cycle are common in Part 2; find a diagram of these events in a standard textbook. The R wave marks the onset of isovolumetric contraction of the left ventricle.

E   Wedge pressure should be read at end-expiration; the QRS complex has nothing to do with it.

XII.27   FTTTT

A,D   In plenum vaporisers, the fresh gas is 'pushed through'. They generally have a high resistance to gas flow, which is one reason why they cannot be used in circuit. Used out of circuit, they can be used with spontaneous breathing.
E   Set at 2% at an ambient pressure of 2 bar, a plenum vaporiser delivers 1% of 2 bar – the same as 2% of 1 bar. Make sure you understand this.

XII.28   TTTTF

The gas laws are not as important in Part 2 as they were in the old Primary. It is not entirely certain at what stage they may be asked (if at all) but it is impossible to understand much of anaesthetic practice (vaporisers, humidifiers, respiratory gas exchange) unless you know about the basic physics of gases.

E   An adiabatic change is one in which temperature changes. The sudden increase in temperature of a rapidly compressed gas can be a fire hazard.

XII.29   TTTTT

E   You should be able to work this out from the Hagen–Poiseuille formula.

XII.30   TTTFF

D,E   Isotopes (for example, hydrogen and deuterium in ordinary and heavy water) can be separated physically because they have different masses, the mass number being the sum of protons and neutrons.

Paper XIII Questions

XIII.1 **In a consideration of acid-base balance:**

  A the buffering power of plasma is greater in vivo than in vitro

  B buffering is greater if the haemoglobin concentration is higher

  C base excess will vary with haemoglobin concentration

  D the normal buffer base is 48 mmol/l

  E the slope of the buffer line increases as buffering decreases.

XIII.2 **Adrenaline:**

  A is synthesised from noradrenaline by a methyl transferase

  B is synthesised from noradrenaline in the adrenal medulla and in nerve endings

  C is metabolised in the liver

  D stimulates glycogenolysis

  E causes systolic and diastolic hypertension when injected intravenously.

XIII.3 ✗ **Important direct factors controlling sodium excretion in the kidney are:**

  A the hydrostatic pressure in peritubular capillaries

  B the rate of tubular secretion of H^+ and K^+

  C aldosterone

  D blood flow in the vasa recta

  E blood pH.

XIII.4 **Pacemaker activity in the myocardium:**

  A can occur in Purkinje fibres

  B is normal in ventricular tissue in vitro

  C starts at the same time as the start of systole

  D starts in the sino-atrial node from a less negative voltage than in other cardiac cells

  E is independent of temperature.

XIII.5 **Serotonin:**

  A is formed by proteolysis

  B causes constriction of skin blood vessels

  C can be metabolised to produce melatonin

  D is present in entero-chromaffin cells

  E is an amide.

XIII.6   The membrane potential of a nerve fibre:

A   represents an imbalance of negative to positive ions on the two sides of a semipermeable membrane

B   can be calculated from the Nernst equation

C   is inversely related to the diameter of the fibre

D   is measured, conventionally, as negative on the inside

E   reverses its polarity during an action potential.

XIII.7   The following are true of normal coagulation mechanisms in vivo:

A   the intrinsic pathway is activated by exposure to vascular endothelium

B   intrinsic pathway activation involves factors XI and XII

C   thrombin is a proteolytic enzyme

D   both intrinsic and extrinsic pathways activate tissue thromboplastin (factor V)

E   thrombin increases platelet aggregation.

XIII.8   The electroencephalogram (EEG):

A   is depressed by anaesthetics in a specific predictable manner

B   is the product of summing many evoked cortical potentials

C   the alpha rhythm is the dominant rhythm in the alert conscious subject

D   the delta rhythm is associated with rapid eye movement (REM) sleep

E   the alpha rhythm frequency is decreased by high $PaCO_2$.

XIII.9   In the regulation of water and sodium:

A   the ascending limb of the loop of Henle is impermeable to water

B   sodium reabsorption from the loop of Henle occurs passively

C   under conditions of maximum antidiuresis, 5% of water reabsorption occurs in the distal tubule

D   anuria is defined as a urine output of less than 0.1 ml/kg/h

E   prolonged thirst induces aldosterone production.

XIII.10 Voluntary hyperventilation for 3 minutes:

A increases arterial carbon dioxide tension
B may cause facial paraesthesiae
C may cause cerebral hypoxia
D decreases arterial oxygen tension
E may cause periodic ventilation on the resumption of normal breathing.

XIII.11 The following are true of the capacity of haemoglobin for oxygen:

A fetal haemoglobin (HbF) has a greater capacity than adult haemoglobin (HbA)
B it is decreased by 2,3-diphosphoglycerate
C under normal conditions it is about 1.35 ml oxygen per gram of haemoglobin
D it is greater than the capacity of myoglobin for oxygen
E it is reduced by carbon monoxide.

XIII.12 Atropine and hyoscine:

A increase the risk of regurgitation
B are contraindicated intravenously in glaucoma
C cause mild neuromuscular blockade in large doses
D are equipotent as drying agents
E produce confusional states.

XIII.13   Phenoxybenzamine:

    A   blocks both α_1- and α_2-receptors
    B   is a non-competitive antagonist
    C   causes reflex tachycardia
    D   reduces supine blood pressure in normal subjects
    E   causes sedation and fatigue.

XIII.14   Protamine:

    A   is a basic protein
    B   1 mg antagonises 100 mg heparin
    C   is a myocardial stimulant
    D   is contraindicated in hepatic failure
    E   is 60% protein bound.

XIII.15   The benzothiazide diuretics:

    A   cause potassium loss
    B   cause loss of bicarbonate relative to chloride ion
    C   block exchange of sodium for hydrogen
    D   have a direct effect on peripheral vascular resistance
    E   cause sodium loss.

XIII.16   Central sedation is a side-effect of:

    A   lignocaine
    B   prochlorperazine
    C   diphenhydramine
    D   atropine
    E   doxapram.

XIII.17   The following are true of isoflurane and enflurane:

    A   they have similar boiling points
    B   isoflurane has the higher molecular weight
    C   they are both contraindicated in anephric patients
    D   adrenaline infiltration is safe
    E   both give measurable fluoride ion in the serum.

XIII.18 **The following pairs of drugs are synergistic:**
- A   penicillin and tetracycline
- B   penicillin and streptomycin
- C   cimetidine and warfarin
- D   tolbutamide and sulphadimidine
- E   atracurium and gentamicin.

XIII.19 **Cocaine:**
- A   causes local anaesthesia by blocking synaptic transmission
- B   potentiates the effects of exogenous catecholamines
- C   is partially hydrolysed by cholinesterase
- D   the maximum permitted dose is about 500 mg
- E   causes mydriasis.

XIII.20 **Plasma cholinesterase activity affects the duration of action of:**
- A   ketamine
- B   edrophonium
- C   vecuronium
- D   suxamethonium
- E   procaine.

XIII.21 **The following drugs cause diarrhoea:**
- A   codeine
- B   neostigmine
- C   atropine
- D   pethidine
- E   carbenoxolone.

XIII.22   The following drugs are chemically steroids:
  A   atracurium
  B   alphaxolone
  C   pancuronium
  D   dexamethasone
  E   propofol.

XIII.23   The following are true of the Wright peak flow meter:
  A   it is a variable orifice flowmeter
  B   rotation of the vane opens a slot for venting of expired gas
  C   the rate and number of rotations of the vane is proportional to peak flow
  D   the peak flow of a fit adult male is 500 l/min or more
  E   the subject makes three attempts at the instrument, the first of which is ignored.

XIII.24   Randomisation of two treatments in a clinical trial means that:
  A   results are treated in random order
  B   treatments are chosen according to unpredictable events occurring within the trial
  C   results are analysed by student's t-test
  D   treatments can be allocated by reference to series of random numbers
  E   treatments are chosen by an independent person.

XIII.25   When recording the electrocardiogram:
  A   the amplitude is usually of the order of millivolts
  B   needle electrodes are safer than plate electrodes
  C   mains interference can be reduced by a screened lead
  D   artefacts caused by muscular tremor can be reduced by a screened lead
  E   the recorded potential is the sum of the individual intracellular action potentials.

XIII.26   The following are true of these vaporisers:
  A   the Boyle's bottle is a plenum vaporiser
  B   the Boyle's bottle has a poor thermal conductivity
  C   back-pressure on a plenum vaporiser may decrease the concentration of vapour in the gas mixture
  D   draw-over vaporisers generally have a lower internal resistance than plenum types
  E   the copper kettle is a draw-over vaporiser.

XIII.27 The pneumotachograph head (Fleisch head):
A measures flow directly
B gives a signal integrated to yield volume
C should be used at room temperature
D must be calibrated for a particular gas mixture
E will give a linear output only over a particular range of flow.

XIII.28 The following measurements alter as increasing clinical concentrations of isoflurane are administered to the patient:
A auditory evoked potentials
B lower oesophageal motility
C train-of-four stimulation
D transthoracic impedance measurement of cardiac output
E pulmonary compliance.

XIII.29 In the measurement of pressure:
A a pressure which supports a 7.5 mm column of mercury will support a 10.2 cm column of water
B 1 kPa is equal to a pressure of 7.5 mmHg
C the mercury column of a sphygmomanometer is closed at the top to prevent contamination and spillage
D a mercury barometer for measuring atmospheric pressure is sealed with a vacuum above the surface of the liquid
E aneroid gauges do not contain liquid.

XIII.30 The following are true of humidity:
A absolute humidity is the mass of water vapour present in a given volume of air
B relative humidity is the ratio of the mass of water vapour present in a given volume of air to the mass required to saturate the same volume of air at the same temperature
C in a hair hygrometer the hair becomes shorter and tighter as humidity increases
D a Regnault's hygrometer contains ether
E the dew point is the temperature at which ambient air is fully saturated.

Paper XIII   Answers

XIII.1   **FTFTF**

   A   There is less buffering power in vivo because of the diffusion of bicarbonate.

   B   Haemoglobin is a very important protein buffer: it has six times the buffering capacity of the plasma proteins.

   C,D,E   Buffer base includes haemoglobin, base excess is independent of it. The steeper the line, the better the buffering. The Siggaard–Andersen nomogram is useful in understanding this.

XIII.2   **TFTTF**

   A,B   Phenyl-ethanolamine N-methyl transferase is found only in the adrenal medulla.

   C   Adrenaline is metabolised in the liver and at the nerve endings.

   E   Classically, because adrenaline has both α and β activity, systolic pressure increases and diastolic pressure decreases, though not as much. The mean pressure therefore increases. The actual effect depends also on the prevailing autonomic tone.

XIII.3   **TTTTF**

   E   Blood pH is not a direct factor; it is a secondary factor, dependent on **B**.

XIII.4   **TFFTF**

   C   The pacemaker potential precedes the action potential.

   D   The lowest potential in the sino-atrial node is about − 60 mV; in other cells it is about − 90 mV. The node cannot strictly be said to have a 'resting' potential.

   E   Pacemaker activity is slowed by hypothermia.

XIII.5   **FTTTF**

   A   Serotonin is synthesised by the hydroxylation and decarboxylation of the essential amino acid tryptophan.

   C   Melotonin is formed in the pineal gland.

   D   Entero-chromaffin cells in the intestinal mucosa secrete serotonin.

   E   Serotonin is an *amine* (5-hydroxytryptamine).

XIII.6   TFFTT

A   The imbalance is extremely small compared with the total number of ions. The imbalance is mainly because K^+ efflux is not accompanied by a corresponding efflux of the protein anions.

B   The membrane potential can be calculated from the Goldman field equation, which contains K^-, Na^+ and Cl^-. The Nernst equation is a general equation for calculating the potential due to a particular ion. The Gibbs–Donnan effect is the effect of non-diffusible protein anions on the distribution of diffusible ions.

C   The potential is independent of the diameter.

XIII.7   FTTFT

You should be able to draw an outline diagram of the coagulation cascade.

A   The blood is normally in contact with the vascular endothelium; the intrinsic pathway is activated by contact with substances exposed by damage to the endothelium, such as collagen.

B   The intrinsic pathway involves factors IX, XI and XII; the extrinsic pathway involves tissue factors, calcium and plasma factor VII.

D   Both pathways activate X, which together with phospholipids and V converts prothrombin to thrombin. However, factor V, an accelerator globulin, does not itself need activation.

XIII.8   FFFFT

A   One of the important problems in anaesthesia is to find a reliable, simple, measurable index of the depth of anaesthesia.

B   The electroencephalogram is a measure of electrical activity in the outermost layers of the grey matter, probably mostly in dendrites, and does not require a stimulus to evoke it.

C   The alpha rhythm is seen at rest: relaxed, and with the eyes closed.

D   The delta rhythm is large slow waves. REM sleep gives a desynchronised, irregular activity.

XIII.9   TFFTT

B   Sodium reabsorption is active from the ascending limb of the loop of Henle, perhaps under the influence of ADH.

C   When conservation of water is maximal, 15% of water reabsorption occurs in the distal tubule

XIII.10   FTTFT

A,D Increased alveolar ventilation will decrease $PaCO_2$ and increase PaO_2 (from the alveolar air equation).

B Facial paraesthesiae is a symptom of reduced ionised calcium.

C Cerebral hypoxia occurs because of cerebral vasoconstriction.

E Hypocapnia causes apnoea, and the periodicity occurs because of a fluctuating hypoxic drive between the periods of reduced ventilation.

XIII.11   FFTTT

The *capacity* is the amount at full saturation. Factors affecting *affinity* do not need consideration.

A HbF and HbA have the same *capacity*

D Myoglobin binds only one mole of oxygen, compared with haemoglobin's four moles, per mole of pigment. Myoglobin's affinity for oxygen is greater than haemoglobin's.

E Carbon monoxide displaces oxygen, and full saturation is not possible.

XIII.12   TFFFF

A That atropine (particularly) reduces the tone of the gastro-oesophageal sphincter is, for some reason, a well-known pharmacological 'fact'. There is no evidence we are aware of that atropine actually increases the incidence of regurgitation. Is the correct answer to this question true or false? It doesn't matter. Most questions do not have these complications; worry about your overall mark, not that you got this one branch wrong.

B *Topical* atropine is contraindicated. The normal intravenous dose, 0.6 mg, will not precipitate glaucoma.

C Neither drug has an effect at the neuromuscular junction.

D Hyoscine is a more potent anti-sialogogue than atropine.

E Both, and especially hyoscine, cross the blood–brain barrier to some extent. They cause confusional states, especially in the elderly.

XIII.13   TTTTT

C,D   *Postural* hypotension is the most troublesome side-effect. There is often a reflex tachycardia, and sometimes other arrhythmias.

E   The fatigue sometimes makes patients too sleepy to eat.

XIII.14   TFFFF

B   1 mg protamine antagonises 1 mg heparin (nominally 100 units).

C   Protamine is a myocardial depressant.

D   There is no contraindication to protamine in hepatic failure.

E   Protamine is highly ionised and protein binding is little.

XIII.15   TFTTT

B   The benzothiazide diuretics cause a relative loss of chloride, hence a hypochloraemic alkalosis.

D   This is true, though the major part of its antihypertensive action is probably by a reduction in blood volume.

XIII.16   TTTFF

A   Although excitation and epileptiform fitting are commonly quoted side-effects of lignocaine, it also has sedative properties and high concentrations cause drowsiness and coma.

C   Diphenhydramine is an antihistamine.

D   Unlike hyoscine, atropine is a central stimulant.

E   Doxapram is an analeptic.

XIII.17   TFFTT

A   The boiling points are isoflurane 58.5°C, and enflurane 56.5°C.

B   They are structural isomers and thus have the *same* molecular weight.

C,E   An anephric patient cannot sustain renal damage. Most anaesthetists would probably avoid enflurane in patients with renal *impairment*, though the plasma concentrations of fluoride ion are not high unless anaesthesia is prolonged. The concentrations of fluoride are even lower with isoflurane, but they are measurable.

XIII.18   TTFTT

Synergism is a specific phenomenon; it does not mean that the drugs interact; or that their effects are similar, or the same, or additive. Synergism means that the drugs together have more than the addition of each individual action.

A,B   These pairs of antibiotics have different spectra and modes of action.

C   Cimetidine may reduce the requirement for warfarin, but this is not synergism because cimetidine is not itself an anticoagulant.

D   Some sulphonamides are hypoglycaemic, for example, sulphanilamide. In fact, these oral hypoglycaemics were discovered by accident during treatment of typhoid fever with sulphonamides, one of the many examples of serendipity in the history of medicine.

E   The combination of an aminoglycoside antibiotic and a non-depolarising neuromuscular blocking drug is synergistic at the neuromuscular junction.

XIII.19   FTTFT

A   Like other clinically useful local anaesthetics the action of cocaine is direct, blocking the transmission of nerve impulses along the axon by blocking sodium channels.

B   Cocaine inhibits re-uptake of noradrenaline at the sympathetic nerve terminal.

C   Cocaine is also hydrolysed in the liver and 10% is excreted unchanged via the kidney.

D   The maximum permitted dose is 100 mg in a 70 kg man.

XIII.20   FFFTT

A   Ketamine is metabolised in the liver by N-demethylation and hydroxylation.

XIII.21   FTFFF

A   Codeine is a constipating drug.

B   Neostigmine increases peristalsis by increasing acetylcholine availability.

C   Atropine is used as an antispasmodic.

D   Pethidine is not a constipating drug, but neither does it cause diarrhoea.

E   Carbenoxolone is an extract of liquorice but it does not cause diarrhoea.

XIII.22   FTTTF

The question asks about drugs that are chemically steroids; it is not asking if they have biological steroid activity.

A   Chemically, atracurium is a bis-quaternary nitrogenous plant derivative

B   Alphaxolone is a steroid anaesthetic, one of the components of the now withdrawn Althesin.

E   Propofol is a hindered phenol.

XIII.23   TTFTF

C   The vane does not rotate completely but only partially, opposed by force from a coiled spring. Do not confuse with the Wright respirometer.

D   The normal value depends on size (it correlates best with height) but more than 500 l/min is an averagely normal figure.

E   The best performance is recorded. Some patients are so breathless that they can manage only one decent blow!

XIII.24   FFFTF

A   The *treatments* are randomised, not the results.

B   This statement is nonsense.

C   That randomisation has been used does not demand any particular statistical test.

D   Random numbers can be looked up from books of statistical tables, or can be generated by computer or hand-held calculator.

XIII.25   TFTFF

B   Needle electrodes carry a higher current density, which risks a greater likelihood of injury if there is an electrical fault.

D   Screening will have no effect on this source of interference. Make sure the patient is comfortable, warm and relaxed.

E   The ECG is the surface expression of intracellular action potentials, and is recorded from only a small area. The sum of the individual action potentials is enormous: 100 mV multiplied by the total number of cells in the myocardium!

XIII.26   TTFTF

C   Back-pressure increases output concentration.

E   The copper kettle is a plenum vaporiser with high thermal conductivity. It is not used clinically but is important theoretically because it delivers a highly accurate concentration of agent.

XIII.27   FTFTT

A,B   The Fleisch head measures nothing directly. It generates a pressure drop that can be measured by manometers, from which the flow is inferred, and volume obtained by integration: flow with time = l/s × s = l.

C   The Fleisch head incorporates a heating coil. Heating prevents condensation of water in the fine tubes. Temperature is thermostatically controlled to ensure the viscosity remains constant.

D   Different gases (or their mixtures) have different viscosities.

E   Heads are calibrated for a given range of flow.

XIII.28   TTFFF

A   Auditory evoked potentials are increasingly delayed as anaesthesia deepens.

B   Oesophageal motility lessens; unfortunately this is not a reliable quantitative measure.

D   Isoflurane reduces blood pressure by decreasing peripheral resistance, but cardiac output remains unchanged (at least at normal *clinical* concentrations). The method of measurement, whether by transthoracic impedance or thermodilution, has no bearing.

E   Isoflurane does not normally affect compliance (although isoflurane may reverse bronchospasm in asthmatic patients).

XIII.29   TTFTT

C,D   The mercury column of a sphygmomanometer, unlike that of a barometer, is open. It measures the gauge pressure above atmospheric.

XIII.30   TTFTT

C   The hair becomes longer.

D,E   The Regnault's hygrometer is used to measure humidity by reference to the saturated vapour pressures at the dew point and at ambient temperature.

Paper XIV   Questions

XIV.1 **Normal electrolyte concentrations in body secretions include:**

A potassium in gastric juice 15 mmol/l
B sodium in bile 30 mmol/l
C sodium in saliva 112 mmol/l
D chloride in gastric juice 140 mmol/l
E bicarbonate in pancreatic juice 10 mmol/l.

XIV.2 **Glucose:**

A has a normal fasting concentration of about 4 mmol/l
B is converted into glucose-6-phosphate by the action of hexokinase
C is converted into glycogen in both skeletal muscle and liver
D is produced enzymically from glycogen in skeletal muscle and liver
E has about the same concentration in plasma and glomerular filtrate.

XIV.3 **Cerebral blood flow is increased by:**

A hypercarbia
B the head down position
C inhalational anaesthetic agents
D sitting up
E sodium nitroprusside.

XIV.4 **Muscle spindles:**

A are receptors which excite the normal reflex arc
B generate afferent impulses carried by fusimotor fibres
C respond to an increase in muscle tension either from active contraction or passive stretch
D contain bundles of modified muscle fibres
E are structures that signal a change in muscle length.

XIV.5 **The secretion of growth hormone is stimulated by:**

A hypoglycaemia
B anaesthesia
C cortisol
D rapid-eye-movement (REM) sleep
E dopamine receptor agonists.

XIV.6 Bile:

 A   secretion is increased by cholecystokinin-pancreozymin
      (CCK-PZ)
 B   is made more acid in the gall bladder
 C   is concentrated up to 40-fold in the gall bladder
 D   contains bilirubin that is mainly unconjugated
 E   is secreted by the parenchymal cells of the liver.

XIV.7 The following immunological phenomena are true:

 A   type 1 immediate hypersensitivity involves IgE
 B   type 2 hypersensitivity binds complement
 C   antigen excess in type 3 produces an Arthus response
 D   delayed hypersensitivity is cell-mediated
 E   cell-mediated hypersensitivity involves complement.

XIV.8 In a consideration of body fluids:

 A   the normal extracellular fluid volume is 15 litres in a 70 kg
      man
 B   total body water is 70% body weight
 C   total body water is simply measured by radioactively
      labelled chloride ions
 D   the volume of interstitial fluid is related to total body
      sodium
 E   the normal daily fluid requirement in the UK is 3 ml/kg/h.

XIV.9 In the glomerulus:

 A   the colloid osmotic pressure is higher in the efferent than
      in the afferent arterioles
 B   the filtration pressure is the difference between the
      hydrostatic pressures in Bowman's capsule and in the
      tubule
 C   molecules up to molecular weight 5000 are filtered freely
 D   molecules of molecular weight over 50 000 are not filtered
      at all
 E   glomerular filtration rate (GFR) is the concentration in the
      urine multiplied by the plasma concentration and divided
      by the urine volume.

XIV.10 When calculating the dead space using the Bohr equation:

 A   arterial and end-tidal samples to estimate the CO_2 are
      equivalent
 B   there must be a steady-state
 C   the assumption is of two 'fractions' in each tidal volume
 D   the result is equivalent to a volume of each breath that
      takes no part in gas exchange
 E   the result is usually expressed at STPD.

XIV.11 √ **Anatomical dead space:**

    A   increases with increasing age
    B   increases in the sitting position
    C   decreases with extension of the neck
    D   is approximately 10 ml/kg body weight in an adult male
    E   is reduced by nasotracheal intubation.

XIV.12 **Intrapleural pressure:**

    A   in quiet respiration is 3–10 cmH_2O below atmospheric pressure
    B   varies during the respiratory cycle
    C   is uninfluenced by positive end-expiratory pressure (PEEP)
    D   is 30–55 cmH_2O above atmospheric pressure on deep inspiration
    E   is less negative at the lung apices.

XIV.13 **These drugs are vasoconstrictors with little or no positive inotropic action:**

    A   adrenaline
    B   methoxamine
    C   isoprenaline
    D   dobutamine
    E   metaraminol.

XIV.14 **Alpha-methyldopa:**

    A   produces a positive Coombs test
    B   causes a negative sodium balance
    C   causes liver damage
    D   results in the formation of a false neurotransmitter
    E   commonly causes sedation.

XIV.15 **Prednisolone is preferred to hydrocortisone in the treatment of inflammation because:**

    A   it causes less gastric irritation
    B   it causes less sodium retention
    C   it does not suppress the secretion of corticotrophin
    D   it has no effect on gluconeogenesis
    E   it is available orally.

XIV.16 **Halothane:**

A   has a saturated vapour pressure of approximately one-third of a standard atmosphere

B   depresses the blood pressure mainly by a direct action on β-adrenergic receptors

C   does not cause respiratory depression until stage III of surgical anaesthesia

D   sensitises the myocardium to the arrhythmogenic actions of catecholamines

E   is contraindicated in jaundiced patients.

XIV.17 **The following are true of the barbiturates:**

A   they were first used clinically in 1941

B   they are readily sequestered in body fat

C   the long-acting drugs, for example phenobarbitone, are excreted unchanged in the urine

D   their distribution in the body is influenced by blood pH

E   the short-acting drugs are largely metabolised in the liver.

XIV.18 **The following local anaesthetic agents are metabolised by pseudocholinesterase:** (ChE)

A   lignocaine

B   procaine

C   amethocaine

D   cinchocaine

E   bupivacaine.

XIV.19 **The following are true in a consideration of intravenous fluid therapy:**

A   0.9% saline contains 140 mmol/l sodium and 140 mmol/l chloride

B   Hartmann's solution contains 8 mmol/l calcium

C   the normal urinary sodium excretion is 70–150 mmol per 24 h

D   the normal urinary potassium excretion is approximately 70 mmol per 24 h

E   the caloric yield of one litre of 20% glucose is 800 kcal.

XIV.20 **Characteristics of neuromuscular blockade by non-depolarising relaxants include:**

A   progressive diminution of the duration of the end-plate potential

B   reduced amplitude of end-plate potential for a given release of acetylcholine

C   synergism between different agents

D   post-tetanic facilitation

E   hypertonus if the patient has myotonia.

XIV.21 Morphine:

A undergoes first-pass metabolism after oral dosage
B remains in the tissues for days
C causes nausea made worse by movement
D causes vasodilatation reversed by naloxone
E causes pinpoint pupils even when tolerance has developed.

XIV.22 Retroperitoneal fibrosis may be produced by:

A chloramphenicol
B ethosuximide
C methysergide
D practolol
E prednisolone.

XIV.23 In the measurement of saturation:

A spectrophotometric measurement in pulse oximetry is made at two points in the infra-red region of the spectrum
B light absorption by oxy- and reduced haemoglobin is equal at the isobestic point
C measurement at the isobestic point provides a reference point independent of haemoglobin concentration
D pulse oximetry readings are falsely low from neonates
E carboxyhaemoglobin interferes with normal pulse oximeter readings.

XIV.24 **When using a flow-directed, balloon-tipped, pulmonary artery catheter (Swan–Ganz):**

    A there is direct measurement of the left atrial pressure
    B once in place the balloon is left inflated to prevent displacement
    C 'wedge' pressure is approximately equal to the left ventricular end-diastolic pressure
    D the volume of the balloon is 5 ml
    E pressures should be measured at end-expiration.

XIV.25 **When considering the uptake of a volatile anaesthetic agent:**

    A the rate of uptake is increased if ventilation increases
    B induction is more rapid if cardiac output decreases
    C induction is less rapid with a less soluble agent
    D the effect of changing cardiac output on the rate of uptake will be greater with a more soluble agent
    E the second-gas effect allows the maintenance concentration of halothane to be reduced when nitrous oxide is used.

XIV.26 **The following methods have been used to assess depth of anaesthesia:**

    A isolated forearm technique
    B sensory evoked potentials
    C lower oesophageal sphincter contractility
    D train-of-four nerve stimulation
    E measurement of thoracic impedance.

XIV.27 **Blood flow:**

    A can be measured ultrasonically
    B as cardiac output may be measured non-invasively by the Fick principle
    C can be measured by variable orifice flowmeter
    D to an organ can be calculated solely from measurements of the washout curve of a radioactive isotope
    E when turbulent results in plasma skimming of blood.

XIV.28 **According to the gas laws:**

    A equal volumes of all gases at the same temperature contain the same number of molecules
    B Avogadro's number is the number of particles in one mole of a substance
    C one mole of any gas at STP occupies 22.4 litres
    D on the gauge of an oxygen cylinder at constant temperature, pressure is proportional to the amount of gas present
    E 42 g nitrous oxide occupies 22.4 litres at STP.

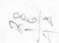

XIV.29 **If a large bubble is connected to a small bubble:**

    A   the pressure in each will be governed by the law of Laplace

    B   the small bubble will empty into the larger one

    C   the addition of a detergent to the system will prevent one bubble emptying into the other

    D   the critical closing pressure is halved

    E   the bubbles will equalise in size.

XIV.30 **At normal room temperature in temperate latitudes, heat loss from the body occurs in the proportion of:**

    A   30% by convection

    B   50% by radiation

    C   10% by evaporation

    D   2% by heating of dry air during respiration

    E   8% by evaporation of water in the respiratory tract.

Paper XIV   Answers

XIV.1   TFTTF

These ionic concentrations in unusual fluids can catch people out. They are important in intensive care if patients are losing large volumes of fluid. **A**, **D** and **E** are more important to know than **B** and **C**.

B   Bile is rich in sodium 145 mmol/l.
E   Pancreatic juice is rich in bicarbonate 110 mmol/l.

XIV.2   TTTFT

B   There is hexokinase in all tissues. The liver also contains the more specific enzyme, glucokinase.
D   Only the liver has the necessary glucose-6-phosphatase to break down glycogen. Otherwise, glycogen is broken down to glucose-1-phosphate by phosphorylase, and in muscle this compound is catabolised via the citric acid cycle or Embden–Meyerhof path.
E   Under normal circumstances, almost all the glucose is reabsorbed.

XIV.3   TTTFF

C and E are pharmacology, and this question is in the physiology section. Questions do occasionally cross-fertilise.

A,C   These cause cerebral vasodilatation.
B   The Trendelenburg position.
E   The effects of nitroprusside on cardiac output are variable. In hypertensive and normotensive patients it has little effect on output; patients in cardiac failure may have improved output. Cerebral blood flow usually remains constant.

XIV.4   TFTTT

B   Fusimotor fibres are gamma motor *efferents*.

XIV.5   TTFFT

C,D   Cortisol and rapid-eye-movement (REM) sleep decrease the secretion of growth hormone.

XIV.6   TTFFT

A   Both CCK-PZ and secretin are responsible for biliary
       secretions.

B,C   Water is absorbed. Bile becomes more concentrated
       and the pH decreases from 8 to 7.2. The percentage
       of solids increases from 2–4% to 10–12% after
       maximal concentration.

D,E   Bilirubin glucuronide, the conjugate, is secreted from
       the liver cells into the bile canaliculi.

XIV.7   TTFTF

C   *Antibody* excess localises the antigen/antibody
       reaction: the Arthus response.

E   This is Type 4, delayed hypersensitivity, and does not
       involve complement.

XIV.8   TTFTF $TBW = 60\%$

C   Total body water is measured using deuterium or
       tritium.

D   The interstitial fluid is a part of the extracellular fluid.
       Sodium, directly and indirectly, is the most important
       regulator.

E   Work it out: 3 ml/kg/h is 5 litres per day.

XIV.9   TFTFF

A   Water and small molecules will have been filtered,
       leaving the proteins behind.

B   There are two active pressures: hydrostatic and colloid
       osmotic pressure.

C,D   There is no absolute cut-off. Hindrance to filtration
       begins above a molecular weight of 5000 and the
       normal kidney should just fail to filter any albumin
       (69 000).

E   The glomerular filtration rate is the urinary
       concentration divided by the plasma concentration,
       multiplied by urine volume (UV/P).

XIV.10   FTTTF

You must know what the Bohr equation is, the assumptions
upon which it is based, and how to derive it: $V_D/V_T =
(P_ACO_2 - P_{\bar{E}}CO_2)/P_ACO_2$ (A is alveolar gas, $\bar{E}$ is mixed
end-tidal).

A   Arterial estimation of carbon dioxide gives the
       physiological dead space, end-tidal the anatomical.

C   The two fractions are the alveolar and the dead space
       fractions; in reality there will be mixing.

E   Usually BTPS or ATPS (which is Ambient Temperature
       Pressure Saturated).

XIV.11   TTFFT

C   Anatomical dead space *increases* on extension of the neck.

D   It is approximately 2 ml/kg.

XIV.12   TTFFF

C   How can this possibly be true?

D   Intrapleural pressure is even more *below* atmospheric than normal during a deep inspiration.

E   Intrapleural pressure is *more* negative at the lung apices.

XIV.13   FTFFT   *Metaraminol - release E, NE ⇒ ? inotrope*

A   Adrenaline is a positive inotrope.

C   Isoprenaline is not a vasoconstrictor.

D   Dobutamine is claimed to increase contractility without affecting rate.

XIV.14   TFTTT

A   One-tenth to one-fifth of patients taking methyldopa long-term develop antibodies that interfere with blood cross-matching.

B   It may cause salt and water *retention*.

C   Hepatitis, jaundice and abnormal liver enzymes have been reported.

D   Its anti-hypertensive action is mainly because it is metabolised to a substance that acts as a false transmitter in the central nervous system.

E   Adverbs of frequency cause problems in MCQs. In **A** and **C** there is no adverb; any described side-effect must then be 'true'. This does not include side effects written up in one-off case reports in obscure journals: use your common sense. Which, if you have read your pharmacology, will tell you that sedation is common with methyldopa.

XIV.15   FTFFF

Prednisolone does cause less sodium retention than hydrocortisone (**B**) but otherwise the two steroids are pretty well equivalent in equipotent dosage. Hydrocortisone is available orally (**E**).

In general, the particular steroid to use can depend as much on the patient as on the indication for use: it is worth reading around this subject.

XIV.16   TFFTF

A   243 mmHg is about one-third of a standard atmosphere (760 mmHg). Remember the SVP does not change with ambient pressure.

B   The hypotensive effect of halothane is mainly by direct myocardial depression, but not via the β-receptors.

C   Respiratory depression is progressive with increasing concentration. This is true for all the commonly used inhalational agents. (Ether is a respiratory stimulant in the lighter stages of anaesthesia.)

E   Do not confuse the jaundice of known cause, in a patient who has not had a recent anaesthetic, with the problems of repeat halothane anaesthesia.

XIV.17   FTTTT

A   Barbiturates were introduced by Fischer and von Mehring, in 1903. The tale of thiopentone at Pearl Harbor (which was 1941) is well known but the drug was introduced commercially in 1935.

C   There is some metabolism of the long-acting drugs but it is very slow, 1% per hour for phenobarbitone.

E   Remember that the *initial* recovery from thiopentone occurs because of redistribution. Metabolism is clinically important in the recovery after methohexitone.

XIV.18   FTTFF

In general, ester-linked local anaesthetics are metabolised by liver and plasma esterases; amide-linked agents are N-demethylated and then hydrolysed) with some urinary elimination.

D   Cinchocaine is no longer available as a local anaesthetic. It is also known as dibucaine, important in the differentiation of abnormal pseudocholinesterases.

XIV.19   FFTTT

A   So-called 'normal' saline contains 150 mmol/l of sodium and of chloride.

B   Hartmann's solution contains 4.4 mmol/l calcium.

XIV.20   TTTTF

C   The interactions between the non-depolarising neuromuscular blocking agents has produced an almost infinite number of combinations for research, but is of limited clinical use.

E   In myotonia, depolarising relaxants may cause hypertonus, but the response to non-depolarisers is normal.

XIV.21 TFTTT

A The effect of an oral dose of morphine is variable, partly because of first-pass metabolism.

B Morphine is cleared fairly rapidly; little remains 24 h after the last dose.

D The vasodilation is only partly because of histamine release.

E Drug addicts have constricted pupils after they have taken the drug.

XIV.22 FFTTF

A Chloramphenicol causes blood dyscrasias.

B Ethosuximide is an anticonvulsant.

C Methysergide is a 5-HT antagonist used for migraine and carcinoid syndrome. It is the drug best known for causing inflammatory fibrosis.

D Practolol was withdrawn from oral use because of retroperitoneal fibrosis.

XIV.23 FTFFT

A Measurements are made at 660 nm (red) and 940 nm (infra-red).

B Note that though this statement is true, pulse oximetry does not make use of the isobestic point.

C Absorbance at the isobestic point varies with the haemoglobin concentration.

D The light extinction curve for fetal haemoglobin is almost the same as that of adult haemoglobin and there will be no error.

E True: the ratio is given by the equation:
$SpO_2 = [(O_2Hb + 0.9 \times COHb)/total Hb] \times 100\%$.
More complex spectrophotometers use more than two wavelengths and can determine COHb and MetHb concentrations.

XIV.24   FFTFT

A,C   The wedge pressure is an indirect pressure transmitted through the pulmonary capillary bed.

B   If the balloon is left inflated there is a risk of distal pulmonary infarction. The balloon is *not* an aid to fixation.

C   'Wedge' pressure is approximately equal to the left ventricular end-diastolic pressure in a normal adult. Part 2 FRCA is a physiology examination, so in general you can assume (unless told otherwise) that questions are about normal physiology, not pathophysiology in patients with chronic pulmonary hypertension.

D   The volume of the balloon is about 1 ml.

E   Pressures are measured at FRC. PEEP or CPAP can make the absolute measurement difficult but for clinical purposes one is usually more interested in changes.

XIV.25   TTFTF

This is an exceedingly important theoretical topic that you must understand, which is why this is the third time of asking.

C   Induction is *more* rapid with a less soluble agent.

E   Second-gas and concentration effects are only of significance in the early induction phase. They are anyway of little practical importance.

XIV.26   TTTFF

The wording is slightly different but this question is virtually the same as XIII.28. If you scored badly at XIII.28, we hope you have read something about the subject in the meantime. You will do better if you know a subject than if you just remember an answer to a specific question.

XIV.27   TTTFF

D   The volume undergoing washout must also be known. Flow is equal to the volume undergoing washout divided by the time constant of the washout curve.

E   Plasma skimming is dependent upon laminar flow occurring at the centre of the vessel.

XIV.28   FTTTF

A   The pressures must also be equal.

E   The molecular weight of nitrous oxide is 44.

XIV.29 TTFFF

A,B,E Pressure is proportional to tension divided by radius. This applies to bubbles (the tension is the surface tension) and also to tubes such as blood vessels (the tension is that in the smooth muscle and elastic tissue).

C An ordinary detergent will merely lower the overall surface tension.

D Critical closing pressure is important in a consideration of the behaviour of small blood vessels and the alveoli. It is, however, out of context here.

B,E These branches are mutually exclusive: questions like this should not be in the exam. Make sure you answered logically – **B** and **E** cannot *both* be right or *both* be wrong, whatever the correct combination is.

XIV.30 TFFTT

B Radiation accounts for 30%.

C Evaporation accounts for 30%.

Paper XV   Questions

XV.1 Acetylcholine acting at muscarinic receptors:
- **A** stimulates adrenaline secretion in the adrenal medulla
- **B** causes vasodilatation
- **C** decreases bronchial tone
- **D** increases ureteric tone
- **E** has prejunctional effects at the neuromuscular junction.

XV.2 The following are consistent with Starling's law of the heart:
- **A** increasing central venous pressure decreases peripheral resistance
- **B** decreasing left ventricular end-diastolic pressure reduces myocardial work
- **C** the energy of contraction is a function of the length of the muscle fibre
- **D** work can be represented by change of ventricular pressure with time (dP/dt)
- **E** increasing afterload decreases cardiac output.

XV.3 The 'blood—brain barrier':
- **A** is the endothelial lining of the arachnoid villi
- **B** is more permeable in the neonate
- **C** does not affect the diffusion of carbon dioxide
- **D** is an active barrier to the diffusion of catecholamines
- **E** is functionally similar to the cell membrane.

XV.4 In the control of thyroid secretion:
- **A** release of thyroid secreting hormone (TSH) is inhibited by a direct feedback loop to the hypothalamus
- **B** there is negative feedback by the thyroid hormones to reduce secretion of TSH by the pituitary
- **C** TSH receptors are linked to a G protein
- **D** TSH has structural similarities to follicle-stimulating hormone
- **E** tri-iodothyronine is more important than thyroxine in feedback regulation.

XV.5 The normal, non-specialised, cell membrane is:
- **A** more permeable to sodium than to potassium
- **B** freely permeable to water
- **C** of low electrical capacity
- **D** freely permeable to mannitol
- **E** more easily penetrated by lipid-soluble than by water-soluble molecules.

XV.6   In the local regulation of the microcirculation:
A   autoregulation occurs in most vascular beds
B   potassium causes vasoconstriction
C   endothelin is an extremely potent vasoconstrictor
D   endothelium-derived relaxing factor is nitric oxide
E   adenosine produces endothelium-independent relaxation of vascular smooth muscle.

XV.7   The pressure of the cerebrospinal fluid:
A   is normally 80–130 mmHg in the lumbar region
B   fluctuates with the blood pressure
C   is generated by CSF being a less effective buffer than plasma
D   alters the rate of its absorption
E   does not normally affect the rate of production of the fluid.

XV.8   The carotid body chemoreceptors:
A   are stimulated by a decrease in arterial oxygen tension
B   are inhibited by a decrease in arterial pH
C   produce reflex peripheral vasoconstriction
D   are responsible for increased ventilation in a patient with carbon monoxide poisoning
E   have a very high tissue blood flow.

XV.9   In the normal pulmonary vascular bed:
A   the mean pulmonary arterial pressure depends on the mean aortic pressure
B   the pulmonary vascular resistance is lower than the systemic vascular resistance
C   there is approximately 1–1.5 litres of blood
D   pulmonary capillary pressure just equals plasma oncotic pressure
E   hypoxia causes reflex vasodilatation.

XV.10   The following are true of normal gastric emptying:
A   fats leave the stomach more slowly than proteins
B   carbohydrates will have left the stomach within 45 min of ingestion
C   increased osmolarity in the duodenum speeds emptying
D   emptying is partly dependent on intact vagus nerves
E   emptying is partly dependent upon the activity of intrinsic factor.

XV.11 Ipratropium:

- A has less effect on the central nervous system than atropine
- B depresses bronchial ciliary action less than atropine
- C is available in inhalers for routine use
- D is of more use in chronic obstructive disease than in asthma
- E does not protect against bronchoconstriction induced by 5-hydroxytryptamine.

XV.12 The following drugs will decrease the mean blood pressure if injected intravenously:

- A phentolamine
- B isoprenaline
- C chlorpropamide
- D thiopentone
- E metoclopramide.

XV.13 Proteinase inhibitors suitable for antagonising fibrinolysis include:

- A streptokinase
- B tranexamic acid
- C stanozolol
- D aprotinin
- E epsilon amino caproic acid.

XV.14 Dextran solutions:

- A may interfere with subsequent cross-matching
- B have useful oxygen-carrying capacity
- C can cause serious anaphylactoid reactions
- D decrease the plasma ionised calcium if infused rapidly
- E may cause acute renal failure.

XV.15 Aspirin-like drugs:

- A reduce prostaglandin biosynthesis
- B act on cyclooxygenase
- C prevent the conversion of arachidonic acid
- D have anti-pyretic activity proportional to their anti-inflammatory activity
- E alter two-point discrimination.

XV.16 The following statements about these inhalational agents are true:

A   methoxyflurane causes polyuric renal failure
B   cyclopropane is explosive with oxygen
C   trichloroethylene is analgesic in subanaesthetic concentrations
D   chloroform increases the likelihood of ventricular arrhythmias
E   chloroform is hepatotoxic.

XV.17 The following statements are true:

A   noradrenaline is a pure α-adrenergic receptor stimulant
B   tetracycline is absorbed better if taken before meals
C   atropine prevents bronchoconstriction caused by cigarette smoking
D   penicillin was the first antibiotic to be used clinically
E   3 mg of atropine will completely block parasympathetic effects on the heart in a normal adult.

XV.18 Prilocaine:

A   is mainly excreted unchanged in the urine
B   is suitable for intravenous (Bier's) block in a 0.5% solution
C   commonly causes methaemoglobinaemia
D   is less likely to cause signs of overdose than lignocaine
E   may produce sleepiness.

XV.19 Ecothiopate is used to treat:

A   glaucoma
B   Eaton–Lambert syndrome
C   hyperhidrosis
D   phenothiazine-induced sedation
E   depression.

XV.20 Release of histamine is a clinical complication in the intravenous use of:

A   streptokinase
B   ranitidine
C   atracurium
D   etomidate
E   gentamicin.

XV.21 Parenteral iron therapy:

A   increases haemoglobin concentration no more rapidly than oral therapy

B   can be given by intramuscular injection

C   may provoke serious anaphylactic reactions

D   is indicated in patients on chronic renal dialysis

E   is indicated in patients receiving total parenteral nutrition.

XV.22 Blood volume:

A   is estimated from red cell volume via measurement of haemoglobin concentration

B   can be measured using labelled albumin

C   can be measured from simultaneous measurement of dilution of labelled sodium and labelled red cells

D   lost during operation can be estimated by haemoglobin dilution in swab washings

E   lost during operation can be estimated most accurately by repeated estimations of haematocrit.

XV.23 A liquid will boil:

A   when its saturated vapour pressure equals atmospheric pressure

B   when its vapour pressure equals its saturated vapour pressure

C   at a higher temperature if it contains a non-volatile solute

D   as its critical pressure is reduced

E   at a higher temperature if the ambient pressure is reduced.

XV.24 For a variable that shows a normal distribution:

A   the median and mean will be the same

B   the variance will equal the standard deviation

C   the sample mean will be equal the population mean

D   the coefficient of variation is a constant

E   a value more than 2 standard deviations from the mean is abnormal.

XV.25 pH = 7.35, PaO_2 = 16.2 kPa (122 mmHg), $PaCO_2$ = 3.5 kPa (26 mmHg) is compatible with:

A   a base excess of – 10 mmol/l

B F_IO_2 = 0.24

C   bicarbonate = 6 mmol/l

D   a partially compensated respiratory acidosis

E   an overcompensated metabolic alkalosis.

XV.26 The following may help prevent electrical injury to the patient in the operating theatre:
    A disconnecting and isolating an external pacemaker
    B a common earth
    C an isolating transformer
    D non-polarising ECG electrodes
    E diathermy held at ground potential.

XV.27 Turbulent flow:
    A is proportional to the square of the pressure
    B is proportional to the length of the tube
    C will become laminar if the radius of the tube is reduced
    D is independent of the viscosity of the fluid
    E is independent of the density of the fluid.

$$\overset{o}{V} = \frac{\partial \sqrt{P}}{Ld}$$

XV.28 The following are true in a consideration of fires and explosions:
    A a stoichiometric mixture is one in which vapour and oxidising agent will be completely used up
    B a stoichiometric mixture carries a maximal risk of explosion
    C isopropyl alcohol 70% in water is not a fire hazard
    D nitrous oxide is capable of supporting combustion
    E the EC (European Community) definition of a zone of risk for the use of flammable gas mixtures is 25 cm from the apparatus.

XV.29 The following devices are used to measure flow:
    A Wright respirometer
    B Benedict–Roth wet spirometer
    C Vitalograph®
    D pneumotachograph
    E dry gas meter.

XV.30 The following aspects of diffusion are true:
    A Fick's law relates rate of diffusion to concentration gradient
    B at tissue level, carbon dioxide equilibration takes 1 s
    C the diffusion rate of available volatile anaesthetics is not an important factor in onset of anaesthesia
    D carbon monoxide is used to measure pulmonary diffusing capacity
    E Graham's law relates the rate of diffusion of a substance to molecular size.

Paper XV   Answers

XV.1   FTFTT

A   The stimulation of the secretion of adrenaline by the
adrenal medulla is a nicotinic action.
C   Acetylcholine increases bronchial tone.
E   The action of acetylcholine at the postjunctional
membrane is nicotinic. There are muscarinic receptors on
the prejunctional membrane, though their function is not
certain.

XV.2   FTTTF

Starling's law is **C**. **B** and **D** are re-statements of it that require
assumptions about the relation of end-diastolic muscle fibre
length to pressure and volume. **A** and **E** may or may not be
true but are not consequent on the law.

Remember that the law can be readily demonstrated in vitro
but in intact animals and man autonomic and other effects
usually override it. Afterload, in particular, is not a useful
measure in intact man.

XV.3   FTTFT

A   The barrier is the capillary endothelium and the choroid
plexus epithelium.
D   All substances cross the barrier to some extent but the
time to equilibration is prolonged compared with transfer
across other capillaries.

XV.4   FTTTT

A   The feedback loop is indirect, via the T3 and T4 released
from the thyroid. Feedback to the pituitary (**B**) is probably
the more important.

XV.5   FTTFT

A   The atomic weight of sodium (23) is less than potassium
(39) and so one might expect sodium to be (in general)
more readily diffusible. However, the hydrated sodium
ion is larger than the hydrated potassium ion.
D   Its use as an osmotic diuretic depends on its not crossing
membranes.

XV.6   TFTTT

In common with much of physiology, now the details of cellular physiology are being worked out, the whole picture is becoming vastly more complicated.

A   We tend to concentrate on autoregulation in the kidney and brain, but most tissues have this ability to some extent.

B   Potassium is vasodilatory.

D   This may sound like a typical 'invented false' answer. As an example of truth being stranger than fiction, it is true: the substance known for some time as EDRF (endothelium-derived relaxing factor) is nitric oxide.

XV.7   FTFTT

A   The figure is correct, but the units should be millimetres of CSF.

C   No, there is not some complex reason why this otherwise perfectly true fact explains CSF pressure: it is nonsense.

D   Absorption is directly proportional to pressure above about 70 mmCSF.

XV.8   TFTFT

B   A decrease in pH is acidaemia, which stimulates the chemoreceptors.

C   This is a reflex caused by stimulation of the chemoreceptors by whatever stimulus, not just hypoxia.

D,E   The blood flow is so high that the oxygen requirements can be supplied by the dissolved oxygen.

XV.9   FTTFF

A,B   The pressure in a system is the product of the cardiac output and the resistance. The pulmonary and systemic systems are separate and controlled independently.

C   The pulmonary circulation contains about one litre, and increases by about 400 ml on lying down.

D   Pulmonary capillary pressure is about 10 mmHg, much less than the plasma oncotic pressure of 25 mmHg.

E   Hypoxia causes vasoconstriction, mainly by a local response.

XV.10   TFFTF

A,B   Carbohydrates leave the stomach most quickly (though not as quickly as 'within 45 min'). Fats leave most slowly.

C   Increased osmolarity in the duodenum *delays* emptying.

E   Intrinsic factor is essential in the absorption of vitamin B_{12}; it has no effect on gastric emptying.

XV.11 TTTTT

B   The lack of effect of ipratropium on ciliary action is an advantage in treating reversible airways disease.

E   This is true; ipratropium is also ineffective against bronchoconstriction induced by leukotrienes, and relatively ineffective against bronchoconstriction induced by histamine, bradykinin or prostaglandin $F_{1\alpha}$. Do not worry if you did not know this.

XV.12 TTFTF

Take care! The important word here is *decrease* the blood pressure; if it were *increase*, the opposite answers would be true. Do not be put off by the question's asking about *mean* blood pressure; systolic and mean pressure usually alter together. An exception is the classic response to isoprenaline, when the β_2 vasodilatation outweighs the β_1 effect on cardiac output.

C   Beware reading this hurriedly as chlorpro*mazine*.

D   We hope you were correct with this one!

E   No effect on blood pressure. You must have the courage of your clinical experience when asked an unexpected question about a common drug.

XV.13 FTFTT

A   Streptokinase is a plasminogen activator.

C   Stanozolol is a testosterone derivative and activates plasminogen. We suspect the correct answer to this branch is 'Don't know'!

D   Trasylol® – a drug that has spent 20 years looking for a disease to treat. At the time of writing it is being used to reduce bleeding in liver transplantation and coronary artery bypass surgery.

XV.14 TFTFT

Dextrans are used less than they used to be; denatured collagen solutions have largely displaced them.

B   None of the blood substitutes currently available carry more oxygen than that in simple solution.

D   There is confusion here with the citrate in blood or plasma infusions.

XV.15 TTTFF

D   All aspirin-like drugs are antipyretic, anti-inflammatory and analgesic, but these three properties differ in relative proportions from drug to drug.

E   The drugs have no effect on any sensation other than pain.

XV.16 TTTTT

A   Detailed knowledge of these agents is no longer
     necessary because they are now of historical interest
     only. **A, B, D,** and **E** are partly the reasons these agents
     are no longer used; **C** was an important property of an
     agent that is sorely missed by those who used it.

XV.17 FTTTT

A   Noradrenaline stimulates β_1 but has little action at β_2.
B   A difficult question. Tetracycline absorption depends
     upon local gastric pH but can be chelated by food, for
     example, calcium in milk.
D   Sulphanilamide was used before penicillin but, not being a
     compound obtained from a living organism, it is not
     strictly an antibiotic although it is an antimicrobial drug.

XV.18 FTTTT

A   Prilocaine is metabolised in the liver, like lignocaine, and
     little reaches the urine.
C   Methaemoglobinaemia is common, but is usually clinically
     unimportant.
D   If procaine is given a safety factor of 1, bupivacaine is
     1.7, lignocaine is 2 and prilocaine is the safest at 3.

XV.19 TFFFF

Ecothiopate is an anticholinesterase that does not cross the
blood–brain barrier. Its only use is the local treatment of
glaucoma. There is a theoretical risk of prolongation of the
action of suxamethonium.

XV.20 TFFFF

There are very few drugs which have not, at some time, been
shown to cause histamine release. What matters is whether
the release is clinically important.
B   Ranitidine is an H_2-antagonist. That does not mean it is
     incapable of causing systemic release of histamine but it
     is not a clinical problem.
C   This is arguable. Local flushing seems common;
     anaphylactoid responses are not.

XV.21   TTTFT
- **A**   Parenteral iron therapy builds up iron stores more rapidly than oral therapy.
- **B**   Intravenous injection is better because of local reactions to intramuscular injection.
- **C**   Intravenous iron is given as iron dextran. The serious anaphylactic reactions that occur are presumably due to the dextran. Careful test doses must always be used and injections made slowly.
- **D**   Patients on chronic renal dialysis absorb oral iron.

XV.22   FFFTF
- **A**   Measuring blood volume by this method requires labelled red blood cells; haemoglobin concentration may vary for many reasons.
- **B**   Using labelled albumin measures *plasma* volume.
- **C**   Labelled sodium measures the total extracellular fluid volume.
- **E**   Measurement of the packed cell volume is often used, but is a rough guide only.

XV.23   TFTFF
- **B**   Saturated vapour pressure *is* the vapour pressure, under the specified condition that the vapour is in equilibrium with its liquid.
- **D**   Critical pressure is a property of the substance and cannot be changed.
- **E**   Boiling point is *lowered* if there is a reduction in ambient pressure.

XV.24   TFFFF
- **B**   The standard deviation is the square root of the variance.
- **C**   The larger is the sample, the better the estimate.
- **D**   The coefficient of variation is the mean divided by the standard deviation.
- **E**   By definition, 5% of normal values lie outside this range.

XV.25   TTFFF
This is a metabolic acidosis with respiratory compensation. The patient must be having oxygen therapy.
- **B**   The maximum PaO_2 with an FIO_2 of 0.24 is about 135 mmHg assuming a normal atmospheric pressure and $PACO_2$.
- **C**   The bicarbonate would be 18 mmol/l.

XV.26 TTTFF

> **B**   There should be a common earth for all electrical
>   equipment attached to the patient.
> **D**   Signal quality will be better with non-polarising electrodes
>   but there is no effect on safety.
> **E**   This is nonsense. The output circuit should be isolated
>   from earth.

XV.27 FFFTF

> You must know the formulae relating flow to pressure and the
> answers to this question follow from them.
> **C**   Reducing the radius will increase velocity and flow will be
>   more likely to be turbulent. If the same flow is directed
>   into many smaller tubes in parallel then the velocity will
>   be unaffected and flow will remain laminar (e.g. the
>   pneumotachograph head).

XV.28 TTFTT

> **C**   Now that inflammable anaesthetic vapours are used
>   rarely, alcoholic solutions for swabbing the skin are the
>   most inflammable compounds in the operating theatre.
>   They have caused some horrific accidents.
> **D**   If the temperature is high enough, nitrous oxide rapidly
>   breaks down to produce a 33% oxygen mixture. This is a
>   theoretical risk if nitrous oxide is used *as the inflating gas*
>   in laparoscopic diathermy.

XV.29 FFFTF

> Of these devices, only the pneumotachograph is used to
> measure flow (and the signal is then integrated electronically to
> give volume). The other devices are used to measure volume.

XV.30 TFTTT

> **B**   Carbon dioxide equilibration is rapid and takes less than
>   0.1 s.
> **C**   Diffusion is rapid enough to be ignored relative to the
>   other factors, such as solubility, ventilation, and cardiac
>   output.
> **E**   Graham's law states that the rate of diffusion of a gas is
>   inversely proportional to the square root of its molecular
>   weight.

Paper XVI Questions

XVI.1 **Adenosine triphosphate:**

    A provides energy for the contraction of skeletal muscle

    B contains two energy-rich phosphate bonds per molecule

    C is synthesised during electron transfer along the flavoprotein–cytochrome system

    D is not produced during the anaerobic metabolism of glucose

    E is hydrolysed enzymatically during the operation of the 'sodium pump'.

XVI.2 **During the normal Valsalva manoeuvre:**

    A there is an initial increase in systolic blood pressure

    B pulse rate increases during the forced expiration

    C there is increased activity of the arterial baroreceptors during the forced expiration

    D peripheral resistance increases during the forced expiration

    E there is a gradual increase of blood pressure back to normal when the glottis is opened.

XVI.3 **Pain:**

    A impulses are transmitted in the lateral spinothalamic tracts

    B is modulated at the spinal level by endorphinergic interneurones

    C is modified at the spinal level by descending fibres from the periaqueductal grey matter of the mid-brain

    D interpretation in the thalamus is inhibited by fibres from the frontal cortex

    E perception requires an intact cerebral cortex.

XVI.4 **Vasopressin:**

    A is a nonapeptide

    B is important in the normal control of blood pressure

    C is inactive by mouth

    D secretion is increased by nausea

    E has a threshold to secretion of about 295 mosmol/l.

XVI.5 **The nerve action potential:**

    A is initiated by potassium efflux

    B is an exponential process

    C can move only in one direction along an axon

    D is propagated by ionic flow through voltage-gated channels

    E is generated by the action of the membrane Na^+-K^+ ATPase.

XVI.6   The complement system:

A   is a system of circulating plasma enzymes
B   is an important mechanism for cell lysis
C   requires previous exposure to the antigen for activation of the alternative pathway
D   includes a number of the clotting factors
E   is a mechanism for the opsonisation of bacteria.

XVI.7 √ Sodium reabsorption in the nephron:

A   is greater in the distal than in the proximal convoluted tubule
B   must be in exchange for other cations to maintain electrochemical balance
C   is the main energy consuming activity of the kidney
D   is the main purpose of the countercurrent multiplier system
E   is dependent on the glomerular filtration rate.

XVI.8   Which of the following are used in the calculation of oxygen availability:

A   cardiac output
B   the oxygen equivalent of haemoglobin
C   physiological shunt
D   the dead-space ratio
E   oxygen saturation.

XVI.9   The effect of surfactant:

A   is to decrease the compliance of the lung
B   is to increase the tissue elasticity of the lung
C   can be estimated experimentally by inflating isolated animal lungs with saline
D   is reduced in pulmonary hypertension
E   is to help keep large airways patent.

XVI.10   The following are true of the respiratory effects of moderate exercise:

A   there is an initial increase of ventilation unrelated to chemical changes
B   increase in ventilation during exercise is proportional to the increase in oxygen uptake
C $PaCO_2$ is little altered during the exercise
D   the hypoxic drive to the peripheral chemoreceptors is an important component in the response
E $PaCO_2$ is increased after the exercise during repayment of the oxygen debt.

XVI.11 **The following statements about β-blockers are true:**

    A labetalol has some intrinsic sympathomimetic activity
    B atenolol is a highly hydrophilic drug
    C esmolol has a half-life of about 30 min
    D timolol used in glaucoma can achieve clinically important plasma concentrations
    E metoprolol undergoes little first-pass metabolism.

XVI.12 **The volume of distribution of a drug:**

    A refers to the peripheral compartment of the two-compartment model
    B makes the assumption that there is a uniform concentration of drug
    C is calculated using the measured concentration in the blood or plasma
    D is affected by differential regional blood flow
    E will be relatively low if hydrophilic and extensively bound to plasma proteins.

XVI.13 **Frusemide:**

    A has its primary site of action in the loop of Henle
    B commonly causes hyperuricaemia
    C enhances the excretion of calcium
    D may induce hyponatraemic acidosis
    E reduces the efficacy of concurrently prescribed lithium.

XVI.14 **The sulphonylureas:**

    A rarely cause hypoglycaemia
    B act mainly by increasing the secretion of insulin
    C are highly protein-bound
    D are safe to use in chronic renal failure
    E are used as a diagnostic test in the incipient diabetic.

XVI.15 Nitrous oxide:

    A is less soluble than oxygen in plasma

    B has sympathetic stimulating properties

    C prevents the effects of carbon dioxide on the cerebral circulation

    D is not a trigger of malignant hyperpyrexia

    E is a potent ventilatory depressant.

XVI.16 In the metabolism of these drugs:

    A morphine forms a conjugated glucuronide

    B penicillin is mainly hydrolysed

    C one of the major metabolic products of halothane is monofluoroacetic acid

    D pethidine metabolism requires catechol-o-methyltransferase

    E cocaine is hydrolysed.

XVI.17 Amino acid solutions for intravenous infusion:

    A are compatible with hypertonic glucose

    B are usually strongly hypertonic

    C contain only essential amino acids

    D are antigenic

    E are buffered by hypophosphate.

XVI.18 The following may potentiate the effect of non-depolarising neuromuscular blocking agents:

    A hypokalaemia

    B hypothermia

    C hypocalcaemia

    D hypermagnesaemia

    E cefuroxime.

XVI.19 Aspirin:

    A may cause iron deficiency anaemia
    B stimulates respiration
    C should not be given to young children
    D causes convulsions in overdose
    E causes tinnitus in overdose.

XVI.20 Convulsions may be produced by:

    A diphenhydramine
    B penicillin
    C phenobarbitone
    D enflurane
    E acetazolamide.

XVI.21 The following are true of flecainide:

    A it is contraindicated in re-entry tachycardias
    B it is a negative inotrope
    C its excretion is slowed in hepatic dysfunction
    D dosage does not need adjustment if renal function is impaired
    E it decreases mortality after myocardial infarction.

XVI.22 The measurement of oxygen content of a blood sample:

    A is not an easy clinical procedure
    B requires haemolysis of the blood sample
    C is affected by the presence of carbon monoxide
    D traditionally is done using the van Slyke apparatus
    E can be done using the Lex-O_2-Con.

XVI.23 The following are normal pressures in a fit adult:

    A aortic root 120/0 mmHg
    B radial artery 130/75 mmHg
    C right ventricle 25/8 mmHg
    D mean end-capillary 17 mmHg
    E mean right atrium 2 cmH$_2$O.

XVI.24   During induction of anaesthesia with a volatile agent:

A   a few deep breaths at the start of induction will ensure the alveolar concentration will equal the inspired concentration

B   the arterial and venous blood concentrations will be the same

C   'overpressure' is possible only with the more volatile agents

D   right-to-left shunts will speed induction

E   left-to-right shunts will speed induction.

XVI.25   Glomerular filtration:

A   is approximately 125 ml/min

B   is influenced by the intrinsic pressure within Bowman's capsule

C   is measured using substances actively secreted into the tubule

D   is reduced in ureteric obstruction

E   has a normal filtration fraction of about 0.2.

XVI.26   In the Severinghaus electrode:

A   the electrode makes contact with sodium bicarbonate solution

B   the electrode is made of CO_2-sensitive glass

C   the plastic membrane is fenestrated to allow the passage of hydrogen ions

D   the electrode works independently of temperature

E   is accurate to $\pm$ 1 mmHg (0.13 kPa) at 40 mmHg (5.3 kPa).

XVI.27   In the electromagnetic spectrum:

A   in air, wavelength is proportional to the reciprocal of the frequency

B   higher frequency implies greater energy

C   the wavelength of ultraviolet is longer than that of infra-red light

D   radio waves have a lower frequency than X-rays

E   gases absorb electromagnetic radiation.

XVI.28 **The following are true:**

A   the application of logarithms will simplify all arithmetic manipulations

B   a logarithmic function is a power function

C   a graphical representation of $y = ax + c$ is a straight line

D   a clinical measurement that is used in monitoring is termed a parameter

E   if the product of two variables is a constant then the relation is hyperbolic.

XVI.29 **Viscosity:**

A   does not affect turbulent flow

B   of blood varies proportionally with the concentration of plasma protein

C   affects blood flow equally in all blood vessels

D   of blood is greater at lower temperatures

E   is measured using a viscometer.

XVI.30 **In the measurement of cardiac output by indicator dilution:**

A   cardiac output is indirectly proportional to the area under the curve

B   using cold as the indicator there is no need to allow for recirculation

C   measurements are accurate to about 5%

D   measurements are less accurate if the haemoglobin concentration is less than 7 g/dl

E   when using indocyanine green sampling can be from any large artery.

Paper XVI   Answers

XVI.1   **TTTFT**
- **B**   Adenosine monophosphate is not a high energy phosphate compound.
- **D**   Anaerobic metabolism of glucose produces fewer ATP molecules per molecule of glucose than aerobic metabolism.

XVI.2   **TTFTF**

The Valsalva manoeuvre is a forced expiration against a closed glottis. It is a common subject for questions in examinations, and rightly so because it is simply explained by knowing the basic principles of cardiovascular physiology. An account of it will be found in any good textbook of physiology.
- **C,D**   The *decreased* activity of the baroreceptors is the afferent limb of the vasomotor reflex to vasoconstriction.
- **E**   The blood pressure overshoots and then decreases to normal.

XVI.3   **TTTTF**

It is helpful to be familiar with a 'circuit diagram' of the proposed mechanism of the gate theory and the transmission and reception of nociceptive stimuli.
- **E**   Argument about this may rapidly become philosophical rather than physiological, but the simple answer for an MCQ is that perception of pain does not need an intact cortex.

XVI.4   **TFTTF**
- **B**   The amount of endogenous vasopressin in the circulation of normal individuals is too small to affect blood pressure.
- **C**   It is frequently given as snuff, absorbed from the nasal mucosa.
- **E**   The threshold to secretion (at least with current methods of detection) is about 280–285 mosmol/l. /kg

XVI.5   **FFFTF**
- **A**   It is initiated by sodium influx.
- **B**   The voltage-gated increase in sodium conductance is rapid, but not exponential, and the process is anyway limited (by the equilibrium potential for sodium).
- **C**   Axons can transmit in both directions, though do not usually do so in vivo.
- **E**   The membrane potential is maintained by the membrane ATPase.

XVI.6   TTFFT

The various components of the complement system are directly or indirectly responsible for many of the consequences of antigen-antibody reactions (including **B** and **E**). The system (of plasma enzymes (**A**)) is separate from the clotting system (**D**), although the two can interact.

C   Previous exposure is required for activation via the classic pathway, but not via the alternative pathway.

XVI.7   FFTFT

A   90% of the sodium is absorbed in the proximal convoluted tubule.

B   There are many transport mechanisms for sodium, not all involve other cations.

D   False — the countercurrent multiplier system renders the medulla hypertonic, and increases the reabsorption of *water*.

XVI.8   TTFFT

'Available oxygen' is a concept for which the cardiac output is multiplied by the total oxygen in the blood, combined and dissolved.

XVI.9   FFFFF

Surfactant *increases* compliance by reducing the forces necessary to overcome surface tension, and it is these forces, not the effect of surfactant, that can be estimated by comparing inflation with saline, which is a measure of elasticity alone, and inflation with air.

XVI.10   TTTFF

The respiratory response to exercise is not fully understood.

A   The initial response is thought to be neural.

D   Hypoxic drive is part of the response, but not an 'important component.'

E   The increased ventilation during repayment of the oxygen debt is caused by lactic acidaemia.

XVI.11   TTFTF

A   This intrinsic activity (at β_2 receptors) may contribute to the vasodilatation.

C   It is not easy to remember exact numbers about drugs, but esmolol is useful *because of* its short half-life, so it is reasonable that users have some idea of how long a dose is likely to last: the quoted half-life is about 8 min.

XVI.12   FTTTT

A,B   The volume of distribution is the volume that would contain a drug at the uniform measured concentration. Neither it, nor the peripheral compartment, has a definable anatomical or physiological volume.

E   This is not always true: if the drug is also largely bound to specific receptors, for instance in muscle, the volume of distribution can be high.

XVI.13   TTTFF

A   The most important site of action is in the ascending limb of the loop of Henle; it also acts on the proximal convoluted tubule.

C   Frusemide is used in symptomatic hypercalcaemia.

D   A good example of when the word 'may' is not a clue that the answer must be 'true'. Frusemide may cause *alkalosis*, often with hyponatraemia.

E   False: frusemide reduces the renal clearance of lithium if there is sodium depletion.

XVI.14   FTTFF

A   All the sulphonylureas can cause hypoglycaemia, especially the longer-acting ones in elderly patients with impaired hepatic or renal function. You could argue about the use of the word 'rarely', but what matters here is whether hypoglycaemia is a danger in a patient who has taken their tablets but no food: it is.

D   Sulphonylureas must be used with caution in renal impairment, especially chlorpropamide because it is not completely metabolised.

E   No, but tolbutamide is sometimes used in the diagnosis of insulinoma.

XVI.15   FTFTF

A   Nitrous oxide is 15 times more soluble than oxygen.
(This question was asked, in reverse, at **V.21**.)

B   Nitrous oxide depresses the contractility of isolated
cardiac muscle but increases circulating noradrenaline
and also increases the responsiveness of vascular
smooth muscle to adrenaline.

C   The effects of carbon dioxide on the cerebral circulation
are unimpaired.

E   Nitrous oxide certainly enhances the depressant effect
of other anaesthetics but could not be itself described
as a potent depressant.

XVI.16   TFFFT

A   The most important pathway for morphine.

B   Penicillin is mainly excreted by the kidneys.

C   There are a number of products, including trifluoroacetic
acid. Cl^- and Br^- are more easily removed from the
halothane molecule than is F^-

D   The interaction here is with monoamine oxidase
inhibitors, which slow the metabolism of pethidine and
can also cause a hyperpyrexic reaction. Pethidine is
hydrolysed, partially conjugated, and also demethylated.

XVI.17   TTFFF

B   The question has to say 'usually' because there are
some preparations that are only slightly hypertonic,
which can be given safely into a peripheral vein.

C   The solutions contain both essential and non-essential
amino acids.

XVI.18   TTTTF

A   An increase in the $[K^+]_i:[K^-]_o$ ratio increases the resting
potential and the amount of transmitter released, which
are conflicting actions. The actual clinical effect is
variable.

B   A complex matter: hypothermia affects many aspects,
physiological and pharmacological, of neuromuscular
transmission.

E   Some antibiotics potentiate the effects of neuromuscular
blocking agents, especially aminoglycosides and
polymyxins, though the clinical effect of a single
intravenous injection is unlikely to cause trouble. This
interaction was a problem with the older blocking
agents when neomycin was used for peritoneal lavage.

XVI.19   TTTTT

A   Iron deficiency anaemia may occur because of continued bleeding from gastric erosions. Calamitous haemorrhage may also occur.

C   Aspirin causes Reye's syndrome in young children. The condition is rare, but paracetamol is a safe, effective alternative.

XVI.20   TTFTF

A   Antihistamines commonly produce drowsiness in overdose but can cause convulsions, especially in children.

B   Convulsions may follow intrathecal injections of penicillin.

E   Acetazolamide is a carbonic anhydrase inhibitor, used as a diuretic and in the prophylaxis of altitude sickness.

XVI.21   FTTFF

A   Re-entry tachycardias (such as Wolff–Parkinson–White syndrome) are an indication for flecainide.

D   The dosage should be decreased in renal failure.

E   In a large well-publicised trial, mortality after myocardial infarction was *increased* by flecainide.

XVI.22   TTFTT

C   The oxygen content will be reduced but measurement is unaffected.

E   The Lex-O$_2$-Con is an important piece of apparatus for the calibration of oxygen measuring devices.

XVI.23   FTFTT

A   This is the left ventricular pressure. Aortic root is 120/80 mmHg.

C   The opposite of **A**: this is pulmonary artery pressure; right ventricle is 25/0 mmHg.

XVI.24   FFFFT

A poor mark here must be rectified by reading and
understanding.

A,B   These situations pertain only at equilibrium, and that is
not practically attainable even with nitrous oxide.

C   Overpressure is possible with all agents except nitrous
oxide.

D,E   The effect of shunts is an extremely complex subject,
further complicated by how the shunt changes as
cardiac output changes with the induction of
anaesthesia. However, other things being equal, a
right-to-left shunt will dilute an inhalational agent, and a
left-to-right shunt will increase its concentration.

XVI.25   TTFTT

C   To measure glomerular filtration rate, the marker must
be neither secreted nor reabsorbed.

D   Back pressure effects.

XVI.26   TFFFT

Candidates at the old Primary FFARCS examination were
expected to know about the Severinghaus electrode in detail.
Quite how much detail is required at the moment is less clear,
but this is an important topic in clinical measurement.

B   It is a modified pH electrode, sensitive to hydrogen
ions.

C   The membrane is permeable to CO_2 but *not* to
hydrogen ions.

D   Temperature must be controlled to $37 \pm 0.1°C$.

XVI.27   TTFTT

C   The wavelength of ultraviolet is *shorter* than that of
infra-red light.

E   This has applications such as infra-red analysis of
carbon dioxide and ultra-violet analysis of volatile
anaesthetics.

XVI.28   FTTFT

Mathematics is important because it can be used to describe so many principles in the basic anaesthetic sciences. We cannot deny that many doctors find mathematics difficult.

A,B Logarithms simplify multiplication or division, by adding or subtracting powers. They are of no help with simple addition or subtraction.

C,D In the equation $y = ax + c$, x and y are variables, while a and c are parameters. This is the correct use of the word parameter (and is correct in statistics because distributions are described by mathematical equations).

E An example is the so-called metabolic hyperbola (CO_2 output $= \dot{V}_A \times PaCO_2$) that results when alveolar ventilation is changed and the resulting $PaCO_2$ measured.

XVI.29   TTFTT

C The effect of viscosity varies with vessel diameter.

E This is the sort of question that sets you wondering in the examination hall: have the examiners really set a question that sounds so easy? Is it a trap? Do not entertain thoughts like these; questions are not set purposely to trap. In viva voce examinations particularly, candidates sometimes go adrift because they simply won't answer the simple question that has been asked but instead try to find a deeper meaning. Usually there isn't one, and the examiner is left with an unfavourable impression. If a more complicated answer is wanted, the examiner will lead you to it – but let the examiner do that job!

XVI.30   TTFFT

A A lower cardiac output causes less dilution, which gives a larger area under the curve.

B Recirculation occurs with the dye indocyanine green, and causes a hump in the exponential decay of the concentration–time curve.

C Thermodilution is accurate to about 20%; dye dilution is better, but only in skilled hands.

D Anaemia does not affect the measurement, though it may affect the cardiac output.

E When cardiac output is measured by indocyanine green, arterial blood is drawn through a spectrophotometer and then re-infused. However, with thermodilution, temperature change will have been dissipated in the tissues long before the sampled blood reaches the artery.

Paper XVII   Questions

XVII.1   **The autonomic nervous system:**
- **A**   is strictly segmented
- **B**   provides the efferent pathway to all viscera
- **C**   comprises all efferent fibres in the body except those to voluntary muscle
- **D**   transmits visceral sensation
- **E**   includes many reflexes integrated in the medulla oblongata.

XVII.2 ✓ **In the fetal circulation:**
- **A**   blood in the ductus arteriosus is more saturated than blood in the ductus venosus
- **B**   blood can pass from the inferior vena cava to the aorta without passing through the heart
- **C**   blood in the umbilical veins is 50% saturated
- **D**   the PaO_2 in the umbilical artery is 2.7 kPa (20 mmHg)
- **E**   blood passing to the brain and arms is better oxygenated than that passing to the lower parts of the body.

XVII.3   **The following statements about electrophysiology are true:**
- **A**   the conduction velocity in the fastest motor fibres in man is $50\,\mathrm{m.s^{-1}}$
- **B**   the resting membrane potential is caused by constant leakage of ions
- **C**   all sympathetic nerves are unmyelinated
- **D**   conduction velocity depends upon local oxygenation
- **E**   axonal conduction is independent of serum magnesium concentrations.

XVII.4   Aldosterone:
A   is formed in the zona reticularis of the adrenal gland
B   has a half-life of 24 h
C   acts on the distal convoluted tubules of the kidney
D   increases the concentration of angiotensin II in the blood
E   is released in response to a high dietary intake of
potassium.

XVII.5   Intraocular pressure:
A   is directly proportional to the blood pressure
B   is increased by coughing
C   is reduced by hyperventilation
D   depends on the angle of the anterior chamber
E   is decreased by osmotic diuretics.

XVII.6   Factors known to enhance fibrinolysis include:
A   menstruation
B   exercise
C   hypercapnia
D   venous occlusion
E   incompatible blood transfusion.

XVII.7   Cerebrospinal fluid:
A   has a specific gravity of 1003–1009
B   has a pH alkaline relative to plasma
C   has a total volume of about 135 ml, of which 25% is in
the spinal space
D   contains no antibodies
E   is produced in a volume of about 550 ml per day.

XVII.8 **Extracellular fluid:**

   A   contains sodium and chloride as the predominant ions
   B   has the same osmotic concentration as sea water
   C   accounts for about 45% of body weight in a normal adult
   D   includes the plasma volume
   E   is a higher proportion of body weight in infancy than in old age.

XVII.9 **In the control of micturition:**

   A   the intravesical pressure increases linearly as the bladder fills
   B   in the period immediately after spinal transection the bladder is flaccid
   C   micturition is initiated by sympathetic nerve impulses transmitted via the ilio-hypogastric nerve
   D   the detrusor muscle can be contracted voluntarily to halt micturition
   E   bladder smooth muscle has inherent contractile activity.

XVII.10 **The central chemoreceptors:**

   A   are more sensitive to changes in the chemical composition of cerebrospinal fluid than of blood
   B   are directly influenced by changes in arterial oxygen content
   C   are located within the respiratory centre of the medulla
   D   respond directly to changes in pH rather than to changes in carbon dioxide tension
   E   are bathed directly by cerebrospinal fluid.

XVII.11 **The oxyhaemoglobin dissociation curve:**

   A   has saturation or content on the y axis
   B   is the graphical representation of the dissociation constant of oxygen
   C   is a reflection of the efficiency of oxygen transport
   D   is represented mathematically by the Hill equation
   E   is hyperbolic if the haemoglobin is in simple solution in plasma.

XVII.12   The Rauwolfia alkaloids:
  A   have been used to treat schizophrenia
  B   interact with intravenous inotropic agents
  C   are a contraindication to β-adrenergic blocking drugs
  D   cause psychological depression
  E   deplete tissue stores of noradrenaline.

XVII.13   Thiazide diuretics decrease blood pressure in the hypertensive patient by:
  A   a mild negative inotropism
  B   a reduction in blood volume
  C   a reduction in vascular tone
  D   a central depressant action
  E   reducing catecholamine re-uptake.

XVII.14   Pharmacological methods of preventing deep venous thrombosis include:
  A   subcutaneous calcium heparin
  B   aspirin
  C   stanozolol
  D   ancrod
  E   streptokinase.

XVII.15   The effects of the following drugs are reversed by naloxone:
  A   thiopentone
  B   methadone
  C   midazolam
  D   pethidine
  E   diamorphine.

XVII.16   Thiopentone has a short duration of action because:
  A   it is metabolised by the liver
  B   it is redistributed to muscle
  C   it is specifically bound to the reticular activating system
  D   it is usually given by rapid intravenous injection
  E   it induces tachyphylaxis.

XVII.17   The possible impurities in commercial nitrous oxide for anaesthetic use are:
  A   ammonium nitrate
  B   nitric oxide
  C   sulphuric acid
  D   carbon monoxide
  E   nitrogen dioxide.

XVII.18   Ether:

A   has a boiling point of 35°C
B   induces upper airway secretions
C   causes progressive bradycardia
D   is contraindicated if adrenaline is to be infiltrated
E   does not cross the placental barrier.

XVII.19   The following are true of chlorpromazine:

A   it has an antipruritic action
B   it is anticholinergic
C   it causes bradycardia
D   it potentiates the ventilatory depression caused by opioids
E   it has a low therapeutic index.

XVII.20   Intravenous lignocaine:

A   depresses pharyngeal reflexes
B   depresses ventilation
C   depresses laryngeal reflexes
D   produces convulsions
E   relieves laryngeal spasm.

XVII.21   Atracurium:

A   is a neuromuscular blocking drug of medium duration of action
B   frequently causes histamine release
C   breakdown by Hofmann elimination depends upon plasma esterases
D   is contraindicated in patients with renal disease
E   laudanum may accumulate in patients receiving prolonged infusions of atracurium.

XVII.22   The following drugs cause local venous thrombophlebitis:

A   methohexitone
B   pancuronium
C   thiopentone
D   etomidate
E   diazepam.

XVII.23   The pneumotachograph:

A   measures directly the pressure change across a resistance
B   has a configuration ensuring laminar gas flow
C   is not suitable for accurate breath-by-breath monitoring
D   has an accuracy affected by changes in temperature
E   has an accuracy unaffected by alterations in gas composition.

XVII.24   The following are true of osmolarity:

A   the depression of freezing point of a solution is proportional to its osmolarity
B   the water vapour pressure of a solution varies with its osmolarity
C   the normal urine osmolarity varies from 300–1400 mosmol/l
D   a urinary osmolarity of 700 corresponds to a specific gravity of 1.040
E   the main determinant of intracellular osmolarity is protein.

XVII.25   The chi-squared test:

A   applies only to continuous variables
B   can prove that one treatment is better than another
C   requires a higher value for chi-squared if the number of degrees of freedom is higher
D   includes a calculation of expected values
E   can only be applied to normal distributions.

XVII.26   Passage of a current through a wire depends on:

A   the resistance of the wire
B   the conductivity of the wire
C   temperature
D   the potential between the ends of the wire
E   the diameter of the wire.

XVII.27   The following are true of diathermy:

A   a high frequency current flows
B   the degree of burning depends upon the current density at the diathermy tip
C   the same current flows through the diathermy tip and the diathermy plate
D   bipolar diathermy does not require a separate plate electrode
E   if the plate becomes detached, the diathermy will not function.

XVII.28 **With a vaporiser 'in circle', the inspired concentration of anaesthetic vapour:**
A   can be less than the nominal concentration
B   can exceed the nominal concentration
C   cannot be altered rapidly
D   increases if minute ventilation increases
E   increases if fresh gas flow increases.

XVII.29 **The following are true of pressure and the units in which it is measured:**
A   pressure is force per unit area
B   the kilopascal is an SI unit of pressure
C   one bar is one standard atmosphere
D   one newton is the force that will give a mass of one gram an acceleration of one metre per second per second
E   surface tension increases the pressure in fine tubes.

XVII.30 **The following mathematical statements are true:**
A   the usual logarithmic base is 2
B 10^{-3} is the reciprocal of 10^3
C   adding the logarithms of numbers is the same as multiplying the original numbers
D   any number raised to the power zero is 1
E   any number raised to the power 1 is the number itself.

Paper XVII Answers

XVII.1 **FTFTT**

A   There is much overlap of segmental innervation in the autonomic nervous system.

C   There are many other efferents, for example fusimotor fibres to muscle spindles.

E   Autonomic reflexes integrated in the medulla oblongata include vomiting, swallowing, and others.

XVII.2 **FFFTT**

Questions about the fetal circulation are asked frequently. You should be able to draw a diagram of the salient features without hesitation.

A   The ductus venosus carries recently oxygenated blood by passage through the placenta. The ductus arteriosus carries blood that is a mixture of oxygenated placental blood and poorly saturated blood from the lower parts of the fetus.

B   Only a small proportion of fetal circulation passes through the lungs, but it all passes through the heart.

C   Blood in the umbilical veins is about 80% saturated in humans.

XVII.3 **FFFTT**

A   The conduction velocity in Aα fibres is 70–120 m.s^{-1}.

B   The membrane potential is generated by the Gibbs–Donnan effect and ionic pumps within the membrane; read about them.

C   Peripheral efferent sympathetic nerves are usually myelinated.

E   Magnesium is an important ion in physiological experiments on nerve conduction and transmission, but it would be difficult to show any effect of physiological changes in serum concentrations. Axonal conduction is certainly unaffected.

XVII.4   FFTFT

A   Aldosterone is formed in the zona glomerulosa. Does it matter? Probably not.

B   It can be difficult to remember figures such as the half-life of hormones exactly ; what is important is to have some idea of the order of things: very short (adrenaline: seconds), short (insulin: 5 min), intermediate (aldosterone: 20 min), very long (thyroxine: 7 d).

C   Aldosterone acts on the distal convoluted tubules and collecting ducts.

D   Aldosterone increases sodium and water retention, so the plasma concentration of angiotensin II is decreased.

XVII.5   FTTFT

A   An increase in systemic blood pressure will be reflected in the intraocular pressure but it is not in direct proportion. Intraocular pressure is modified by local homeostatic mechanisms.

C   Hyperventilation probably reduces intraocular pressure, at least at first, because hypocapnia causes vasoconstriction. Excessive hyperventilation might, however, increase intraocular pressure by raising the venous pressure.

D   Glaucoma is more likely if the angle is narrow, but pressure then increases because of blockage of the canal of Schlemm.

XVII.6   TTTTT

XVII.7   TFFTT

B   Some authorities hold that the pH of cerebrospinal fluid and plasma is the same in the steady-state; others that cerebrospinal fluid is the more acid (pH of 7.33, compared with 7.40). It is not more alkaline. Buffering and the interrelations of the acid-base balance of plasma and CSF is a complex subject.

C   Total volume is about 150 ml, 75 ml is in the spinal space. Questions that ask if a figure is correct must give a value well outside the normal range for it to be wrong.

E   The turnover of cerebrospinal fluid is about 3.7 times a day.

XVII.8   TFFTT

B   Although the ECF is sometimes spoken of as the 'internal sea', sea-water is actually hypertonic.

C   Do not make the mistake of incorrect association: 45 is the number of litres of total body water in the normal 70 kg adult. Extracellular fluid makes up 20% of body weight in the adult.

D   Plasma volume is 5% of body weight and interstitial fluid 15%.

XVII.9   FTFFT

A   The smooth muscle of the bladder has the property of plasticity: when stretched, the initial tension is not maintained. Intravesical pressure remains low until the bladder contains about 400 ml urine.

B,E   The bladder is flaccid in spinal shock. Inherent tone later returns in paraplegic patients.

C   The sympathetic nerve supply to the bladder is not involved in micturition.

D   The detrusor muscle is the smooth muscle of the bladder wall and increases intravesical pressure.

XVII.10   TFFTF

B   The central chemoreceptors do not respond to hypoxia. They are depressed in extreme hypoxia, as is most of the central nervous system. They are affected indirectly by hypoxia because of changes in cerebral blood flow.

C   The central chemoreceptors are separate from the respiratory centre.

E   The receptors are thought to be a little way beneath the surface.

XVII.11   TFFTF

B,C   These branches are meaningless. It is easy to be seduced by scientific sounding explanations, but you *know* what the oxyhaemoglobin dissociation curve is: it relates the saturation of haemoglobin to the partial pressure of oxygen. A common response to this kind of question is to answer 'Don't know'. If you have done enough work for the examination you should have the knowledge to recognise these branches for the red herrings they are.

E   The sigmoid shape is because of the effect of 2,3-DPG in the red cells.

XVII.12   TTFTT

The Rauwolfia alkaloids are now used rarely for the treatment of hypertension but they are important theoretically because of their interactions at the adrenergic nerve terminal; to understand these interactions helps understanding of the processes at the terminals.

XVII.13   FTTFF

There are many thiazide diuretics but none has any advantage over bendrofluazide, except that chlorthalidone has a longer duration of action and allows prescription on alternate days.

    A   Beware of being tempted to answer 'true' because of the word 'mild'.

XVII.14   TTFTF

    C   Stanozolol is a derivative of testosterone. It is a plasminogen activator indicated for the treatment of the vascular manifestations of Behçet's disease, but not for the prevention or treatment of deep venous thrombosis

    D   Ancrod is a preparation of a snake venom that prevents polymerisation of fibrin. The drug had some popularity for a time. You must get used to the fact that there will be some questions about which you will not have a clue; as long as there are not too many it does not matter and you must not worry about them.

    E   Streptokinase is a plasminogen activator used to stimulate fibrinolysis when there is established clot.

XVII.15   FTFTT

Naloxone is a specific opioid antagonist. There are no specific antagonists to barbiturates; flumazenil is an antagonist to benzodiazepines.

XVII.16   FTFTF

    A,B   Thiopentone is metabolised slowly. The rapid initial recovery is because of redistribution to muscle; redistribution to fat is a slower process.

    D   There will not be rapid recovery after a thiopentone infusion.

XVII.17   FTFFT

    A   Nitrous oxide is manufactured by heating ammonium nitrate, but it is a solid and will not be found as a contaminant.

XVII.18   TTFFF

Ether is important historically and because it is still used in some parts of the world.

C   Increased sympathetic tone causes tachycardia.
E   All anaesthetic agents cross the placental barrier readily.

XVII.19   TTFTF

C   Chlorpromazine may cause tachycardia secondary to some α-adrenergic blockade.
E   Coming after **C** and **D**, both of which are side-effects, there is the temptation to answer 'true': it has side-effects – therefore it must have a low therapeutic index. But the answer is 'false'; the phenothiazines are safe agents that can be given safely over a wide range of dosage.

XVII.20   TFTTT

B   Lignocaine is not a specific respiratory depressant even in excess.

XVII.21   TFFFF

B   Histamine release does sometimes occur, but not 'frequently'.
C   Hofmann elimination is a non-enzymatic process. Some atracurium is broken down by plasma esterases, but the two processes are unconnected.
D   Atracurium can be completely metabolised in the plasma and does not require hepatic or renal function.
E   Read the question! Laudan*um* is a term for tincture of opium; the metabolite of atracurium is laudan*osine*. A trick question perhaps, but patients have died because of confusion over drug names.

XVII.22   FFTTT

A,C   At the usual dilutions, thiopentone (2.5%) is more likely to cause thrombophlebitis than methohexitone (1%).
D   Etomidate causes thrombophlebitis in up to 30% of patients. The incidence depends on the solvent.
E   The high incidence of venous thrombophlebitis caused by diazepam led to its reformulation in Intralipid® as Diazemuls®.

XVII.23   TTFTF

C   The pneumotachograph is designed for this purpose.
E   Changes in gas composition affect viscosity and density separately, and therefore alter accuracy because there must be laminar flow and whether flow is laminar depends upon both viscosity and density.

XVII.24   TTTFF

D   A urinary osmolarity of 700 corresponds to specific gravity 1.020.
E   The main determinant of intracellular osmolarity is potassium.

XVII.25   FFTTF

A   The chi-squared test applies to occurrences, though they may be of continuous variables: the blood pressure being above or below a certain value in a comparison of different conditions.
B   Statistics cannot prove treatments are better (or worse) than others. All they do is place a mathematical probability on the observed differences having occurred by chance.
C   Have a look at a table of the chi-squared distribution.
E   The chi-squared test is a non-parametric test; it does not depend on the distribution of the data. There are tests (for example, the Student's 't' test) that strictly should only be applied to data that conform to the normal distribution.

XVII.26   TTTTT

A,B,E   Conductivity is the reciprocal of resistance. For a given material, resistance varies with the inverse of diameter.
C   The dependence of current on temperature is important in the thermocouple.

XVII.27   TTTTF

A   The frequency is MHz.
E   The diathermy will function (unless the machine has safety features to prevent it, which most modern machines do). The circuit will be completed by the route of lowest electrical resistance and may cause burns.

XVII.28   **FTFTF**

A,B   Recirculation means that the inspired concentration must be at least equal to the nominal concentration.

E   Fresh gas in the circuit dilutes the anaesthetic vapour.

XVII.29   **TTFFF**

B   *The* SI unit of pressure is the pascal; the prefix is an SI prefix.

C   One bar is 10^5 N.m^{-2} (100 kPa). The standard atmosphere is 760 mmHg, or 101.315 kPa, which is 1013 millibar. The bar is not an SI unit.

D   One newton gives a mass of one *kilo*gram an acceleration of 1 m.s^{-2}.

E   Surface tension causes a *misreading* of pressure if a column of fluid is read in a fine tube.

XVII.30   **FTTTT**

A   The usual bases are e (so-called natural logarithms) and 10.

Paper XVIII   Questions

XVIII.1   **Iron absorption:**
   A   is usually about 15 mg per day
   B   is regulated according to body stores
   C   takes place in the terminal ileum
   D   includes a stage of storing in the intestinal cells in combination with apoferritin
   E   is increased by a high phosphate concentration in the diet.

XVIII.2   **The venous return:**
   A   is increased by a deep inspiration
   B   is increased on first assuming the upright posture
   C   is unaffected by arteriovenous fistulae
   D   decreases in moderate exercise
   E   is regulated directly by aldosterone.

XVIII.3   **Unilateral damage to the cerebellum in man produces:**
   A   disturbances of posture
   B   no difficulty initiating voluntary movement
   C   intellectual impairment
   D   uncoordinated movement only when the eyes are closed
   E   ipsilateral loss of position sense.

XVIII.4   The thyroid hormones:
A   are synthesised from alanine
B   are active in the L-form
C   are highly bound to plasma proteins
D   are partly bound to albumin
E   have calorigenic actions modulated by circulating catecholamines.

XVIII.5   The following gastric secretions are essential to life:
A   hydrochloric acid
B   intrinsic factor
C   pepsin
D   rennin
E   gastrin.

XVIII.6   Factors which predispose to the development of a hypersensitivity reaction to an intravenous anaesthetic induction agent include:
A   atopy
B   infection
C   previous exposure to the agent
D   the formation of precipitates by drug interaction within the intravenous cannula
E   preoperative hypovolaemia.

XVIII.7   In excitation–contraction coupling in skeletal muscle:
A   acetylcholine spreads from the neuromuscular junction into the T tubules
B   calcium is released from the sarcoplasmic reticulum
C   calcium binds to troponin C
D   tropomyosin is formed by the complexing of actin and myosin
E   the energy is obtained directly from ATP.

XVIII.8   The following measurements are consistent with physiological oliguria:
A   urine sodium less than 10 mmol/l
B   urine specific gravity greater than 1.024
C   a urine:plasma osmolarity ratio of 5:1
D   a urine:plasma urea ratio of 100:1
E   a urine:plasma creatinine ratio of 20:1.

une urine : plasma osm 2.5 : 1
une plasma creat 60 : 1
une plasma urea 100 : 1

XVIII.9   For a group of alveoli that are under-ventilated but which have normal perfusion:

- A   the PaO_2 will be less than normal
- B   the $PaCO_2$ will be less than normal
- C   the $\dot{V}/\dot{Q}$ ratio will be less than normal
- D   the saturation of blood in those pulmonary arterioles will be less than normal
- E   the effect on overall $PaCO_2$ will be less than on overall PaO_2.

XVIII.10   In the normal pulmonary circulation:

- A   capillary pressure is about 10 mmHg
- B   angiotensin II is inactivated
- C $PGF_{2\alpha}$ causes vasoconstriction
- D   the velocity of blood in the root of the pulmonary artery is the same as that in the aorta
- E   of the fetus, about 15% of the cardiac output goes to the lungs.

XVIII.11   Alveolar minute ventilation:

- A   is equal to total minute ventilation minus the dead space ventilation
- B   can be calculated from the alveolar air equation
- C   is equal to tidal volume multiplied by respiratory rate
- D   is about 4.5 l/min at rest
- E   varies with posture.

XVIII.12   In acute hepatic failure:

- A   blood clotting is impaired
- B   serum alkaline phosphatase can be normal
- C   serum albumin may be less than 10 g/l
- D   the bromsulphthalein excretion test is valid only in the absence of jaundice
- E   serum lactic dehydrogenase is a sensitive index of hepatocellular damage.

XVIII.13   Alpha-adrenergic blockade is produced by:

- A   phentolamine
- B   isoprenaline
- C   labetalol
- D   indoramin
- E   phenylephrine.

XVIII.14   Digoxin:

    A   increases the contractile force of the normal human heart

    B   dilates arteriolar and venous beds in the forearms of normal subjects

    C   produces an increase in serum potassium

    D   makes electrical defibrillation of the heart less certain

    E   dosage should be increased in hypothyroidism.

XVIII.15   Hypokalaemia occurs with:

    A   triamterene

    B   carbenoxolone sodium

    C   frusemide

    D   spironolactone

    E   ammonium chloride.

XVIII.16   Metformin:

    A   does not cause the lactic acidosis sometimes seen with phenformin

    B   does not cause hypoglycaemia in normal subjects

    C   should not be given with a sulphonylurea

    D   is ineffective unless there are functioning islet cells

    E   is contraindicated in the alcoholic patient.

XVIII.17   The following are true in a consideration of the mechanism of general anaesthesia:

    A   the potency of volatile anaesthetics is related to their lipid solubility

    B   pressure reversal applies only to volatile anaesthetics

    C   MAC correlates best with lipid solubility

    D   the narcotic potential of inert gases and vapours is inversely proportional to their vapour pressures

    E   there is a theory related to the formation of hydrate microcrystals.

XVIII.18 **In the excretion of these drugs:**
  A   about 25% of phenobarbitone is excreted unchanged in the urine
  B   phenothiazines are excreted conjugated with glucuronic acid
  C   at least 60–80% of halothane is excreted through the lungs
  D   neostigmine is excreted unchanged
  E   gallamine is excreted mainly via the liver.

XVIII.19 **Tinnitus is caused by:**
  A   codeine
  B   aspirin
  C   cocaine
  D   tobramycin
  E   amphetamine.

XVIII.20 **Suxamethonium:**
  A   increases intraocular pressure
  B   decomposes rapidly in solution if not stored at 4°C
  C   should not be used in patients who have sustained severe burns
  D   increases serum potassium in normal patients
  E   causes muscle pains more likely in ambulant patients.

XVIII.21 **Dependence occurs in patients treated with:**
  A   methadone
  B   phenoperidine
  C   buprenorphine
  D   naloxone
  E   pentazocine.

XVIII.22 **Ketorolac trometamol :**
  A   has marked anti-inflammatory properties at analgesic doses
  B   reduces patient requirements for opioid drugs
  C   alters protein binding of digoxin
  D   should be given in reduced dosage to patients with renal impairment
  E   is contraindicated in patients who are allergic to aspirin.

XVIII.23 The following can be used to test recovery from anaesthesia:

A   p deletion test
B   sensory evoked potentials
C   Maddox wing test
D   flicker fusion test
E   spectral edge analysis.

XVIII.24 Functional residual capacity:

A   is increased when lying down
B   is about 3 litres in a normal young man
C   can be measured by a nitrogen washout technique
D   is increased in pregnancy
E   can be measured by plethysmography.

XVIII.25 The following statements about the effects of gaseous anaesthetic agents are true:

A   the second gas effect is produced by rapid diffusion of large volumes of nitrous oxide into the blood
B   the displacement of oxygen from the alveoli by nitrous oxide during recovery from anaesthesia is known as diffusion hypoxia
C   an increase in cardiac output during anaesthetic induction will decrease the alveolar concentration of nitrous oxide
D   the alveolar concentration of a very volatile and very soluble anaesthetic agent increases more rapidly if ventilation is depressed
E   the concentration effect results in more rapid equilibration between alveolar and inspired concentrations.

XVIII.26 The fidelity of the reading from a trace of direct arterial pressure will be improved if:

A   an incompressible fluid completely fills the system
B   the system has a resonant frequency equal to the pulse rate
C   the transducer has a diaphragm of high compliance
D   the catheter is made of stiff material
E   a long catheter of narrow bore is used.

XVIII.27 Boyle's law:

A   describes the relation between the volume and pressure of a gas
B   is independent of the mass of the gas
C   applies only at constant temperature
D   applies to all gases and vapours
E   is incorporated in the universal gas law.

XVIII.28 **The following are true of Rotameters®:**

A they are variable orifice flowmeters
B the pressure across the bobbin remains constant
C at high flows, the increase in area of the annular orifice reduces resistance
D flow is laminar over the calibrated portion of the tube
E they must be vertical for accurate readings.

XVIII.29 **Intra-operative heat loss is minimised by:**

A increasing the ambient theatre temperature
B using a local anaesthetic technique
C covering the patient with a plasticised sheet
D placing the patient on a warming mattress
E using an airway heat and moisture exchanger (HME).

XVIII.30 **Techniques suitable for sterilisation of a fibreoptic laryngoscope include:**

A washing with chlorhexidine
B low temperature autoclaving
C gas sterilisation with ethylene oxide
D soaking in glutaraldehyde
E soaking in ethyl alcohol.

Paper XVIII   Answers

XVIII.1   **FTFTF**

A   *Intake* may be 15 mg, of which 3–6% will be *absorbed.*

B   The amount of transferrin in the bloodstream is inversely proportional to the amount of iron in the body. Greater saturation of transferrin leads to reduced uptake from the mucosal cells.

C   Iron absorption occurs in the upper small intestine.

E   Phosphate balance is linked with calcium, not iron.

XVIII.2   **TFFFF**

A   A deep inspiration increases the pressure gradient from the great veins to the thoracic cavity.

B   We don't talk about 'assuming the upright posture'; we talk about 'standing up'. Medical language is full of these pomposities, and that includes examination papers. Standing reduces venous return, for hydrostatic reasons, though compensation is rapid in normal subjects.

C   Where else can the shunted blood go?

D   Exercise increases cardiac output, so venous return must increase.

E   Aldosterone acts indirectly, via sodium balance and extracellular fluid volume.

XVIII.3   **TTFFT**

Questions on neurological damage are not uncommon, even though the examination is in physiology; understanding neurological function is often best explained by what happens when nerve pathways are damaged.

B,C   Cerebellar damage may cause some difficulty with voluntary movement, but not with the initiation of the movement (which occurs in parkinsonism); nor does it cause intellectual impairment.

D   Incoordination is not worsened by closing the eyes, unlike in tabes dorsalis.

XVIII.4   FTTTT

A   The thyroid hormones are synthesised from tyrosine. When two molecules of di-iodotyrosine condense to form T_4, a molecule of alanine is eliminated.

B   Yes: the L-forms are 300 times more active than the D-forms.

D   Thyroid hormones are bound 12% to albumin, and 88% to thyroxine-binding globulin.

E   The calorigenic effect of a single injection of thyroxine depends upon the level of catecholamine secretion and the metabolic rate before injection. If the initial metabolic rate is low, the calorigenic effect is great; if it is high, the calorigenic effect is small.

XVIII.5   FFFFF

Think what one needs to replace after gastrectomy.

B   It is vitamin B_{12}, not intrinsic factor, that is essential and given as replacement therapy after gastrectomy.

C   It is actually pepsinogen that is secreted, but it is not essential.

D   Rennin is probably not produced in humans.

XVIII.6   TFTTF

A   All reactions are more likely in atopic individuals, irrespective of prior exposure.

D   Some immunologists are more convinced by the 'immune-complex' theory than others, but in the current state of knowledge this answer is true: they may predispose towards hypersensitivity reactions.

E   Preoperative hypovolaemia may worsen the resulting hypotension, but does not make a hypersensitivity reaction more likely.

XVIII.7   FTTFT

A   Depolarisation spreads electrically into the T tubules.

D   Tropomyosin, which prevents interaction between actin and myosin when the muscle is relaxed, moves when calcium is bound to troponin C, allowing interaction.

XVIII.8   TTFTF

C,E   A urine:plasma osmolarity ratio of 2.5:1 and a urine:plasma creatinine ratio of greater than 60:1 are consistent with physiological oliguria.

XVIII.9   TFTFF

Underventilation and normal perfusion is a low $\dot{V}/\dot{Q}$ ratio (C), the normal state at the base of the lung.

A,B P_AO_2 will be less than normal and P_ACO_2 will be greater than normal.

D   This is the blood *supplying* the alveoli.

E   This is the classic error in understanding gas exchange. That there is usually less effect on P_ACO_2 is because of the shape of the oxyhaemoglobin dissociation curve, not because of diffusibility. Find someone to help you understand this.

XVIII.10   TFTTT

B   Angiotensin I is converted to angiotensin II, which is unaffected by passage through the lung.

D   Velocity depends on flow and cross-sectional area of the blood vessel, not on pressure.

XVIII.11   TFFTT

B $P_AO_2 = P_IO_2 - P_ACO_2/RQ$. The alveolar air equation allows calculation of the partial pressure of oxygen in the alveoli; it has nothing to do with ventilation.

C   This cannot be true: tidal volume includes the dead space volume.

XVIII.12   TTFTF

C   In severe hepatic disease, albumin may be 20–25 g/l.

E   Skeletal and heart muscle, and red blood cells, also contain lactic dehydrogenase. The enzyme is insensitive as a specific index of hepatic disease.

XVIII.13   TFTTF

B,E   Isoprenaline is a β-agonist; phenylephrine is an α-agonist.

XVIII.14   TFFTF

B   Digoxin has no effect on peripheral vasculature.

C   Careful! The link between digoxin and serum potassium is that hypokalaemia makes arrhythmias more likely. If anything, the improvement in renal blood flow consequent on better cardiac function would increase potassium *loss*, not cause an increase in the serum concentration.

E   The risk of toxicity is increased in hypothyroidism.

XVIII.15   FTTFF

A,D   Triamterene and spironolactone (an aldosterone antagonist) are potassium-conserving diuretics; *hyper*kalaemia is a risk.

E   Ammonium chloride is an acidifying diuretic: two moles produce one mole of urea (which is an osmotic diuretic) and one mole of hydrogen ions.

XVIII.16   FTFTT

A   Metformin is less likely than phenformin to cause lactic acidosis.

C   Combined therapy with sulphonylureas is not contraindicated, but patients may become hypoglycaemic so blood glucose should be monitored.

D   Metformin reduces absorption of carbohydrates from the gut and aids peripheral utilisation of glucose.

E   Lactic acidosis is more likely in alcoholics.

XVIII.17   TFTTT

A,C   The link with lipid solubility is the Meyer–Overton theory, probably the best known of all the ideas of how general anaesthesia works, and dating from 1899–1901.

B   Pressure reversal occurs with all anaesthetics.

E   The hydrate microcrystal theory (the formation of 'clathrates') is due to Pauling.

XVIII.18   TTTFF

B   In general, do not guess at MCQs. However, this might be an exception: most chemically complex drugs are, at least partly, inactivated by conjugation with glucuronic acid and the resulting water-soluble conjugate is excreted in the urine.

D   Neostigmine is hydrolysed by plasma esterases and then excreted in the urine.

E   Gallamine is not used much nowadays, but was well known as a drug whose main route of elimination is the kidney. Prolonged paralysis occurred in patients with impaired renal function.

XVIII.19   FTFTF

B   Tinnitus is a recognised symptom of aspirin poisoning.

D   The aminoglycoside antibiotics cause VIIIth nerve damage if given in overdose, especially to patients with renal failure. Tinnitus is one sign of this damage.

XVIII.20   TFTTT

A   Suxamethonium does increase intraocular pressure, but the increase is transient (and there is much argument about whether it matters).

B   The solution deteriorates in hot conditions and ampoules are best kept in a refrigerator, but the answer here is 'false'.

C   To 'should *not* be used' the answer is 'true'. 'Should *never* be used' could generate much discussion.

XVIII.21   TTTFT

Some drugs are more addictive than others, but (to the continuing chagrin of drug companies who think they have at last found the non-addictive opioid) all opioids are addictive.

XVIII.22   FTFTT

A   Ketorolac has little anti-inflammatory action at analgesic doses.

C   Ketorolac *is* protein bound in the plasma, but it is a highly potent drug which is present only in low concentrations.

XVIII.23 TFTTF

B,E   Sensory evoked potentials and spectral edge analysis (of the electroencephalogram) are under investigation to assess depth of anaesthesia but are not useful at assessing whether a patient has recovered from the effects of anaesthetic drugs.

XVIII.24 FFTFT

A,D   Functional residual capacity is decreased when lying down or in pregnancy.

B   The volume of the functional residual capacity depends on sex and height. It is just more than 2 litres in the 'normal young man'.

XVIII.25 TTTFT

C   The effect of cardiac output on alveolar concentration is greater with a soluble agent. For an insoluble agent such as nitrous oxide, cardiac output will have virtually no effect after the induction phase.

D   Do not be distracted by the extra details: the alveolar concentration of *any* inhaled anaesthetic is *decreased* if ventilation is depressed.

XVIII.26 TFFTF

The word fidelity is the same as in hi-fi meaning high-fidelity: does the electrical signal (from the pressure transducer or loudspeakers) reproduce the pressure wave (from the artery or the orchestra) accurately?

Fidelity covers not just the accuracy of the systolic and diastolic pressures but the shape of the waveform as well. You must know in outline about natural frequency, damping and critical damping. Do not try to learn the mathematics of frequency response unless you are good with equations and figures.

B   If the system has a resonant frequency equal to the pulse rate, the whole thing resonates ('rings'). The systolic pressure over-reads, and the signal develops false secondary peaks.

C   The diaphragm should be stiff: of *low* compliance.

XVIII.27 TFTFT

B   Boyle's law describes a given mass of gas.

D   Strictly Boyle's law applies only to ideal gases; practically, it applies to all gases unless close to liquefying. There is no rigid difference between a gas and a vapour: a vapour above its critical temperature is a gas.

XVIII.28   TTTFT

B	The force balances the force of gravity on the bobbin.
D	Flow is laminar in the lower part but turbulent in the upper part.
E	There are inclined plane flowmeters, but Rotameters® must be read vertically.

XVIII.29   TFTTT

B	Local anaesthetic techniques do not affect heat loss directly; some, such as epidural anaesthesia, may increase heat loss by affecting autonomic control of the circulation.

XVIII.30   FFTTF

A,E	Neither chlorhexidine nor ethyl alcohol kills bacterial spores.
B	Putting a fibrescope in an autoclave would cause expensive damage.
C	Gas sterilisation with ethylene oxide is effective but not many hospitals have the facility.
D	Glutaraldehyde requires special precautions; sterilisation must be done in a washer or fume cupboard.

Paper XIX   Questions

XIX.1   **Mammalian genes:**
  A   are segments of DNA
  B   contain untranslated segments known as introns
  C   are transferred into the cytoplasm for expression as proteins
  D   are the same in all somatic cells of a given species
  E   give rise to messenger-RNA by the process of transcription.

XIX.2   **In the metabolism of carbohydrates:**
  A   the phosphorylation of glucose to glucose-6-phosphate by hexokinase is a reversible reaction
  B   5% of ingested glucose is converted to liver glycogen
  C   there is a paradoxical increase in blood glucose in starvation
  D   fat is readily converted to glucose
  E   glucagon increases blood glucose by an effect on liver phosphorylase.

XIX.3   **Oxygen consumption by cardiac muscle:**
  A   increases in exercise by a much increased coronary blood flow
  B   increases in exercise by a much increased oxygen extraction
  C   is regulated at the cellular level by cardiac myoglobin
  D   is directly correlated with ventricular work
  E   is increased more by the demands of increased pressure than by equivalent increases in volume.

XIX.4   **Damage to the main sensory area of the brain produces:**
  A   little loss in sensation to pain
  B   limb rigidity
  C   unconsciousness
  D   marked loss of the sensation of fine touch
  E   cortical blindness.

XIX.5   **The following are true of the thyroid hormones:**
  A   thyroxine (T_4) is the most active natural compound
  B   more than 99% of active hormone is protein-bound
  C   their actions are mediated via receptors on the cell surface
  D   an increase in metabolic rate occurs within minutes of increased hormone activity
  E   they increase the number of cardiac β-adrenoceptors.

XIX.6   In the stomach:

A   there is approximately 3 litres of gastric secretion per day
B   the parasympathetic innervation is from the coeliac plexus
C   gastric emptying is controlled by periodic relaxations of
     the pyloric sphincter
D   catecholamines inhibit secretion
E   the contents are normally sterile.

XIX.7   The withdrawal reflex:

A   is a polysynaptic reflex
B   can be demonstrated by stretching a muscle beyond the
     length at which the stretch reflex is exhibited
C   involves more limbs as the stimulus increases
D   is faster if the higher centres are intact
E   is an example of a mass reflex.

XIX.8   The following are true of the triple response:

A   it is part of the normal response to injury
B   the first part is the white reaction
C   the flare is caused by arteriolar dilatation
D   the weal is absent in sympathetic denervation
E   there is evidence it is an axon reflex.

XIX.9   In a fit, healthy subject breathing 100% oxygen:

A P_AO_2 = 90 kPa (675 mmHg)
B PaO_2 = 85 kPa (637 mmHg)
C CaO_2 = 21.5 ml per 100 ml
D PvO_2 = 7 kPa (52 mmHg)
E   raising the ambient pressure does not increase oxygen
     content.

XIX.10   In exercising skeletal muscle:

A   maximum oxygen uptake is not limited by blood flow to
     the muscle
B   venous PO_2 increases
C   unitary oxygen extraction increases up to 30-fold
D   the onset of fatigue is unrelated to oxygen extraction
E   tissue pH decreases.

XIX.11 In sodium balance:
  A   the normal daily sodium requirement is 70–140 mmol
  B   the normal daily sodium intake is 10–15 g
  C   sodium is actively absorbed in the small intestine
  D   exchangeable sodium is more than 90% of total body
      sodium
  E   resting intracellular sodium concentration is 5–10 mmol/l.

XIX.12 Side effects of ganglion blocking drugs include:
  A   ileus
  B   atony of the bladder
  C   postural hypotension
  D   miosis
  E   bradycardia.

XIX.13 Amiodarone:
  A   is a class IB anti-arrhythmic drug
  B   does not cause clinically important myocardial depression
  C   is unlikely to cause side-effects if trouble-free for the first
      3 months of treatment
  D   can cause pulmonary toxicity
  E   interferes with tests of thyroid function.

XIX.14 Diclofenac:
  A   does not inhibit platelet function
  B   is poorly absorbed when taken orally
  C   has a prolonged plasma half-life relative to other
      non-steroidal drugs
  D   is excreted mostly unchanged in the urine
  E   is especially suitable in the third term of pregnancy.

XIX.15 The following are true of steroid therapy:
  A   hydrocortisone replacement alone is sufficient in Addison's
      disease
  B   dexamethasone is suitable for replacement therapy
  C   methylprednisolone is a more potent anti-inflammatory
      agent than hydrocortisone
  D   prolonged steroid therapy may cause osteoporosis
  E   cortisone does not cause fluid retention.

XIX.16 Etomidate:
  A   has no muscle-relaxing properties
  B   inhibits adrenal steroidogenesis
  C   increases the tone of pharyngeal muscles
  D   does not cause hypotension on induction of anaesthesia
  E   produces a low incidence of allergic-type reactions.

XIX.17 The following drug interactions occur:

    A phenobarbitone can decrease the effect of phenytoin

    B potassium potentiates the action of digitalis

    C coumarin anticoagulants increase the hypoglycaemic effect of tolbutamide

    D tamoxifen increases the speed of onset of non-depolarising neuromuscular blocking agents

    E cimetidine decreases the bioavailability of propranolol.

XIX.18 Tachyphylaxis may be a problem during short-term treatment with:

    A ephedrine

    B trimetaphan

    C suxamethonium

    D noradrenaline

    E sodium nitroprusside.

XIX.19 Acetylcholinesterase:

    A is present in plasma

    B is inhibited by pilocarpine

    C will hydrolyse dibucaine

    D is present in high concentrations in the placenta

    E hydrolyses acetylcholine faster than other choline esters.

XIX.20 Glycopyrronium:

    A is a quaternary amine

    B is a more effective anti-sialogogue than atropine

    C is an effective anti-emetic

    D causes less tachycardia than atropine

    E is less sedating than hyoscine.

XIX.21 In digoxin overdose:

    A there are pathognomonic arrhythmias

    B there is anorexia

    C toxicity may be increased by hypokalaemia

    D toxicity may be increased by hypocalcaemia

    E arrhythmias may be treated with propranolol.

XIX.22 Acyclovir:

A   is a general inhibitor of viral replication
B   is active when taken by mouth
C   is active topically against herpes simplex infections
D   is usually well tolerated by intravenous infusion
E   causes encephalopathy.

XIX.23 Cyclosporin:

A   is a selective inhibitor of T-cell activation
B   is dependent on the cytochrome P_{450} system for its clearance
C   is nephrotoxic
D   suppresses bone marrow
E   causes pulmonary fibrosis.

XIX.24 The measurement of carbon dioxide in breathing systems in the operating theatre:

A   is commonly by infra-red absorption
B   is more accurate with in-line sensing than with a side-stream sensor
C   under-estimates end-expired carbon dioxide at high ventilatory rates
D   requires in-built electrical compensation for water vapour
E   is not affected by high clinical concentrations of volatile anaesthetic agents.

XIX.25 Uptake of inhalational anaesthetic agents from the alveoli into the blood depends upon:

A   alveolar concentration of the agent
B   blood solubility of the agent
C   cardiac output
D   body temperature
E   ventilation/perfusion ratio.

XIX.26 The partition coefficient:

A   relates the ratio of amounts of a given substance between two phases
B   for gases, can be expressed as the ratio of the partial pressures between two phases
C   is affected by temperature
D   is affected by atmospheric pressure
E   is defined at equilibrium.

XIX.27   Saturated vapour pressure:

    A is dependent on the ambient pressure

    B increases linearly with ambient temperature

    C is the pressure exerted at equilibrium by a vapour in contact with its liquid

    D of water at body temperature is 6.3 kPa (47 mmHg)

    E can be estimated from the molecular weight by using Henry's law.

XIX.28   In the constant flow of gas along a tube:

    A the pressure is a reflection of potential energy

    B the velocity is a reflection of the kinetic energy

    C the Venturi effect depends on the Bernoulli principle

    D turbulent flow has a flat velocity profile

    E flow through an orifice within the tube is dependent only on the size of orifice if the pressure drop is high.

XIX.29   In a bobbin flowmeter such as the Rotameter®:

    A viscosity of the gas is important in calibration at low flows

    B density of the gas is important in calibration at low flows

    C the area around the bobbin behaves as an orifice at high flows

    D electrostatic forces are most likely to cause the bobbin is to stick at the top of the tube

    E bobbins are interchangeable between flowmeter tubes.

XIX.30   In a consideration of pressure:

    A a wider bore syringe can generate a higher pressure

    B the pressure required to open an expiratory valve at its minimum setting is approximately 1.5 cm water

    C the pressure in a full oxygen cylinder is approximately 138 atmospheres

    D the pressure in a nitrous oxide cylinder depends on the size of cylinder

    E gauge pressure is measured value plus atmospheric pressure.

Paper XIX Answers

XIX.1 **TTFTT**
  B Segments of genes are exons, which are translated, and introns, whose function is uncertain.
  C The DNA of the genes does not leave the nucleus.

XIX.2 **FTFFT**
  A Glucose is converted to glucose-6-phosphate by hexokinase, but a different enzyme (the liver enzyme glucose-6-phosphatase) catalyses the reverse reaction.
  C There is a slight *decrease* of blood glucose in starvation.
  D Glucose can be converted to fats via pyruvate and acetyl-CoA, but this reaction is irreversible and there is little conversion of fat back to glucose.

XIX.3 **TFFTT**
  B Oxygen extraction is almost maximal in the coronary circulation all the time.
  C This is a typical false answer: sounds plausible, but nonsense.

XIX.4 **TFFTF**
  B,C Neither limb rigidity nor unconsciousness occurs with damage to the sensory cortex. There may be incoordination of an affected limb.
  E Cortical blindness occurs with damage to the occipital (visual) cortex.

XIX.5 **FTFFT**
  A Thyroxine is, to a large extent, a pro-compound to the more active tri-iodothyronine.
  C Thyroid hormones are transported into cells and bind to the nuclei.
  D Metabolic rate increases within hours, not minutes.

XIX.6   TFFTT
B   The parasympathetic innervation is from the vagus; the
        sympathetic innervation is from the coeliac plexus.
C   The pylorus is not important in the regulation of gastric
        emptying.

XIX.7   TFTFF
The withdrawal reflex is the motor response to a nociceptive
stimulus.
B   This is the inverse stretch reflex, for which the afferent
        is the Golgi tendon organ.
C   The full response is difficult to demonstrate in an intact
        animal but can be seen in the spinal preparation – or in
        a patient with a severe spinal or head injury.
D   This is false, although the speed of a polysynaptic
        reflex, unlike a monosynaptic reflex, can vary.
E   This is false, although the withdrawal reflex is *part of*
        the mass reflex (the exaggerated neural response seen
        in chronic paraplegic patients).

XIX.8   TFTFT
B,D   The triple response is red reaction, weal, flare. It is the
        response to firm pressure from a pointed object. The
        white reaction is the response to light pressure from a
        pointed object. The response is a local one that
        depends upon the integrity of the *local* sensory nerves.

XIX.9   TTTTF
A,B,D   These figures are approximate, but are in the correct
        range.
C   This figure is correct for the 'normal' concentration of
        haemoglobin, which, as a single figure, can be taken as
        15 g/dl.
E   The higher the ambient pressure, the more oxygen will
        dissolve.

XIX.10   TFFTT
B,C   Venous PO_2 decreases as unitary oxygen extraction
        increases about three-fold (this contrasts with cardiac
        muscle, see **XIX.3**). Muscle blood flow increases about
        30-fold. Oxygen delivery thus increases 90-fold.
D   Fatigue in exercise is ill understood.

XIX.11   TTTFT

C   Sodium also diffuses passively, in or out depending on the gradient.

D   Exchangeable sodium is 65–70% of total body sodium.

XIX.12   TTTFF

D   Ganglion blocking drugs dilate the pupils (mydriasis).

E   There will be (variable) reflex tachycardia, due perhaps to parasympathetic blockade or to the baroreceptor reflex.

XIX.13   FTFTT

A   The I–IV classification system is well known (though somewhat confusing). Amiodarone is a class III drug.

C   Adverse effects are particularly likely if treatment is prolonged.

XIX.14   FFFFF

A   All non-steroidal anti-inflammatory drugs alter platelet function.

B   Diclofenac is well absorbed.

C   Diclofenac does not have a prolonged half-life but it does accumulate in synovial fluid, which may explain its prolonged effect at this site.

D   These drugs are mostly metabolised or conjugated.

E   Diclofenac is not recommended for pregnant women (though few new drugs are).

XIX.15   FFTTF

A   Fludrocortisone must be given as well.

B   Dexamethasone has little mineralocorticoid activity. It is used mainly in suppression tests and as a potent anti-inflammatory agent.

XIX.16   TTFFT

D   Etomidate has less cardiovascular effect than the other commonly used induction agents, but it is not true to say that *it does not cause hypotension*.

XIX.17 TFTFT

A   This apparent paradox arises because phenobarbitone
        induces microsomal enzymes, which increases the
        metabolism of drugs given concurrently.
B   No: hypokalaemia increases the likelihood of digoxin
        toxicity.
C   There is competition between tolbutamide and warfarin
        for binding sites on plasma proteins.
D   More and more women are likely to be taking
        tamoxifen. There are no known interactions with any
        of the drugs used in anaesthesia.

XIX.18 TTTFT

Tachyphylaxis often occurs with indirectly acting pressor
drugs. The effect of a directly acting pressor may become
less with time during longer treatment, because of
down-regulation of the receptors. This is not what was meant
originally by the term tachyphylaxis, which is confusing.
C   Probably linked with the change from phase 1 to phase
        2 block that occurs with repeated doses.

XIX.19 FFFTT

A   At the neuromuscular junction, and in the CNS.
B   Pilocarpine is a cholinomimetic used in glaucoma.
C   The confusion here is that dibucaine (cinchocaine) will
        inhibit the action of plasma cholinesterase and is used
        in the diagnosis and differentiation of atypical
        cholinesterase.
E   It is also one of the most efficient enzymes known.

XIX.20 TTFFT

C   Hyoscine is the only one of this group of drugs that is
        used as an anti-emetic.

XIX.21 FTTFT

A   *Pathognomonic* means a symptom or sign from which,
        of itself, the disease or condition can be diagnosed.
        Just about any arrhythmia can occur in digoxin toxicity,
        and none is specific to it.
C,D   No: by *hyper*calcaemia. Potassium and calcium
        frequently have opposing effects.
E   Phenytoin, lignocaine and potassium are the most
        effective (but don't give potassium if it was high
        initially). Quinidine, procainamide and propranolol are
        sometimes effective but frequently produce new
        arrhythmias.

XIX.22   FTTTT

A   Acyclovir is useful only in herpes infections. This is
        because it has particular affinity for herpes-encoded
        thymidine kinase, which is not a fact that anaesthetists
        are expected to remember, though its consequence is
        clinically important.

XIX.23   TTTFF

B   This is important because any drug that induces
        hepatic enzymes can reduce the concentration of
        cyclosporin enough to cause rejection.
C   Decreasing renal function because of cyclosporin
        toxicity has to be differentiated from decreasing
        function secondary to rejection.
D   An advantage of cyclosporin is that it does not
        depress the marrow.
E   Pulmonary fibrosis has not been reported.

XIX.24   TFTFT

B   Side-stream analysis may introduce a slight delay but is
        not less accurate.
C   At respiratory rates approaching 30 the response time
        of the systems may not be fast enough to give true
        peak and trough readings.
D   Side-stream capnographs have water traps to prevent
        drops of water forming in the sensing cell.

XIX.25   TTTTT

There are few excuses for getting anything other than five out
of five for this question if you have worked through this book.

XIX.26   TFTFT

B,E   The partition coefficient is the ratio of amounts
        between two phases at equilibrium (which means the
        partial pressure of a gas will be the same in both
        phases) where the phases are of equal volume.
D   Atmospheric pressure does not affect partition
        coefficient, though it will affect the *total amount* of
        atmospheric gases dissolved in a phase exposed to
        them.

XIX.27   FFTTF

A   A basic principle that you must understand is that saturated vapour pressure depends on the temperature and the nature of the liquid *only*.

B   It is an approximately exponential relation, which is different for each liquid.

E   There is no way of estimating saturated vapour pressure from molecular weight, and Henry's law governs the solubility of a gas in a liquid.

XIX.28   TTTTT

E   This is the so-called 'critical orifice', used in gas mixing devices.

XIX.29   TFTFF

A,B,C Flow around the bobbin is laminar at low flows and turbulent (the annulus around the bobbin behaves like an orifice) at high flows.

D   Electrostatic sticking is more likely at the bottom of the tube where it is narrower. There may be a spring at the top of the tube to stop the bobbin jamming at the top after excessive gas flows.

E   Each tube and bobbin are calibrated together for a specific gas and are inaccurate for other gases of different viscosity or density.

XIX.30   TTTFF

A   Pressure is force per unit area. A wider bore syringe will generate a lower pressure.

E   Gauge pressure is zero when a cylinder is 'empty', and the contents are then at one atmosphere pressure.

Paper XX Questions

XX.1 **The following statements about the autonomic nervous system are true:**

A there are cell bodies of preganglionic neurones in the motor nuclei of cranial nerves

B there are cell bodies of preganglionic neurones in the dorsal root ganglia

C preganglionic axons are mostly myelinated

D sympathetic postganglionic neurones lie mostly in the tissue of the innervated organs

E the parasympathetic division has no outflow from the thoracic segments.

XX.2 **Blood volume:**

A is partly regulated by erythropoietin

B is independent of the extracellular fluid volume

C is increased by salt loading

D can be measured by a dilution technique using labelled red cells

E returns to normal within 24 h of a loss of 20% of the initial volume.

XX.3 **In neurophysiology, the term 'all-or-none' means that:**

A monosynaptic reflexes are involved

B the amplitude of a propagated action potential is independent of the size of the stimulus

C transmission cannot occur unless all the synaptic receptors are activated

D recruitment does not apply

E there will be a refractory period.

XX.4 **Parathyroid hormone:**

A mobilises calcium from bone

B increases tubular reabsorption of phosphate

C is a polypeptide

D is regulated by calmodulin

E is secreted by the chief cells.

XX.5 **In the neonate:**

A the tidal volume is 17–19 ml

B the mean blood pressure is 65 mmHg

C about 20% of the haemoglobin is haemoglobin A

D the PaO_2 is a little higher than in the adult

E the ductus arteriosus constricts gradually over the 24–48 hours after delivery.

XX.6 Prostaglandins:

A are eicosanoids
B increase renal cortical blood flow
C are metabolised in the pulmonary circulation
D modulate the action of histamine and bradykinin in pain
E are stored in mast cells.

XX.7 The following pairings of visceral organs and segmental innervations for pain are correct:

A the heart and aorta via T1–T5
B the adrenals via T9–T12
C the uterus via T11–L2
D the urinary bladder via T11–L2.
E the gall bladder via T4–T10.

XX.8 There are peripheral chemoreceptors:

A in the carotid bodies
B supplied by the glossopharyngeal nerve
C in the adrenal medulla
D in the aortic arch
E in the right atrium.

XX.9 The diffusion capacity of the lung:

A can be measured by uptake of carbon monoxide
B can be measured by uptake of nitrous oxide
C can be measured by uptake of oxygen
D is increased in exercise
E varies with lung compliance.

XX.10 The following are consequences of the shape of the oxyhaemoglobin dissociation curve:

A oxygen uptake in the lungs is little affected by small changes in P_AO_2
B oxygen delivery in the tissues can be large for small changes in partial pressure
C the affinity of haemoglobin for oxygen increases with partial oxygenation
D there is a good diffusion gradient for oxygen in the lung
E oxygen affinity is altered by altered $PaCO_2$.

XX.11 In the passing of a chemical message across cell membranes:
 A neurotransmitters bind to membrane G-proteins
 B adenylate cyclase is activated by G-proteins
 C down regulation is a decrease in the number of receptors
 D guanosine triphosphate combines with the α subunit of a G-protein
 E the acetylcholine receptor at the neuromuscular junction is a voltage-gated channel.

XX.12 Glyceryl trinitrate is an effective treatment for angina because:
 A the threshold of cardiac pain receptors is raised
 B there is reflex bradycardia
 C there is improved coronary perfusion
 D afterload is reduced
 E blood volume is reduced.

XX.13 The following are true of oral iron therapy:
 A a measurable increase in haematocrit should occur within 7–10 days of the start of treatment
 B treatment can usefully continue even after the haemoglobin concentration has become normal
 C ferrous salts are the most effective preparations
 D gastro-intestinal side-effects are rare
 E symptoms of overdose include hyperventilation due to metabolic acidosis.

XX.14 Metoclopramide:
 A blocks central dopamine receptors
 B antagonises the emetic action of ergotamine
 C does not cross into breast milk
 D has a prolonged half-life in patients with renal failure
 E is effective in high intravenous doses for the emesis of cancer chemotherapy.

XX.15 Ketamine hydrochloride:
 A is an arylcycloalkylamine
 B increases pulmonary vascular resistance
 C increases myocardial contractility in vivo
 D has bronchodilatory properties
 E increases tone in skeletal muscles.

XX.16 Ethanol (ethyl alcohol):
- A is a stimulant of the central nervous system
- B depresses the ventilatory response to carbon dioxide
- C causes cutaneous vasodilatation
- D is metabolised by first-order kinetics
- E is a poor source of energy.

XX.17 Effects of chlorpromazine include:
- A α-adrenergic blockade
- B antihistaminic action
- C hypothermia
- D constipation
- E miosis.

XX.18 Absorption of local anaesthetics from tissues depends upon:
- A tissue solubility of the agent
- B vascularity of the tissue
- C concentration of the drug
- D rate of breakdown by tissue esterases
- E local pH.

XX.19 Vecuronium:
- A is metabolised in the liver
- B is metabolised by pseudocholinesterase
- C blocks noradrenaline re-uptake by nerve terminals
- D does not cause bronchospasm
- E is contraindicated in renal failure.

XX.20 Naloxone:
- A is a μ-receptor antagonist
- B is an analogue of morphine
- C is a respiratory stimulant in normal man
- D reverses the analgesic effects of placebo
- E has a duration of action of one to four hours.

XX.21 If pethidine is given to a patient receiving monoamine oxidase inhibitors the following may occur:
- A hypotension
- B ocular palsies
- C coma
- D Cheyne–Stokes respiration
- E cerebral excitation.

XX.22 Zidovudine (AZT):

- **A** is active against HIV-1
- **B** treatment is started by intravenous infusion
- **C** rarely causes marrow depression
- **D** causes acute neurotoxicity
- **E** toxicity is increased by aspirin.

XX.23 Streptokinase:

- **A** is obtained from β-haemolytic streptococci
- **B** binds with plasminogen to form plasmin
- **C** will not cause bleeding in the absence of intravascular thrombus
- **D** is contraindicated in patients with a history of scarlet fever
- **E** may cause a pyrexia.

XX.24 If a large sample (n = 200) has a normal distribution:

- **A** the arithmetic and geometric sample means will be the same
- **B** about 96% of the observations will be within two standard deviations of the mean
- **C** the population mean will be within the 95% confidence interval of the sample mean
- **D** bias is unlikely
- **E** the z-ratio can be used to compare means with a second large sample.

XX.25 The mass spectrometer:

- **A** is so named because of its ability to distinguish molecules within a mixture of molecules
- **B** detects ionised particles
- **C** has a response time fast enough for breath-to-breath measurements
- **D** cannot be used for molecules made up of more than three atoms
- **E** is useful for small samples.

XX.26 The following statements about electricity are true:

A the standard calibration on an ECG monitor is 1 mV = 1 cm on the screen

B the frequency of alternating current in Britain is 60 Hz

C the peak voltage of alternating current in Britain is 340 V

D Ohm's law states that current flowing in a circuit is directly proportional to the voltage and inversely to the resistance

E impedance depends on the frequency of the current.

XX.27 In a defibrillator:

A at maximum setting a potential of thousands of volts is applied across the capacitor plates

B energy stored is dependent upon charge and potential applied

C if 400 joules are released the current pulse will be of the order of 35 amperes for 3 ms

D the energy required for internal defibrillation is approximately 100 joules

E when synchronised defibrillation is used, the energy is discharged synchronously with the P wave of the ECG.

XX.28 Entonox:

A is supplied in a cylinder with a blue and white shoulder

B has the same saturated vapour pressure as nitrous oxide at a given temperature

C should be stored at temperatures higher than 10°C

D is 50% oxygen and 50% nitrous oxide

E supports combustion.

XX.29 The following are true of the solubility of gases:

A Henry's law states that the gas dissolved is directly proportional to the partial pressure of the gas

B as a liquid is warmed less gas is dissolved in it

C solubility of a gas depends on the surface tension of the liquid

D the Bunsen solubility coefficient is for one standard atmosphere pressure of the gas

E the Ostwald solubility coefficient is independent of ambient pressure.

XX.30 The latent heat of vaporisation of a liquid:

A decreases with an increase in temperature

B is maximal at its critical temperature

C causes cooling as the liquid evaporates

D prevents the freezing of the liquid

E is zero at the liquid's boiling point.

Paper XX Answers

XX.1 **TFTFT**

Autonomic anatomy and physiology are important. These are basic questions that you should have answered correctly. If you did not, you should look at a textbook.

XX.2 **FFTTF**

A Erythropoietin affects red cell production and maturation, not blood volume.

B The plasma component of the blood volume is part of the extracellular fluid volume.

D Red cells can be labelled with ^{51}Cr. Other techniques use albumin labelled with isotopes of iodine.

E It takes 12–72 h to restore the circulating plasma volume. Initially the tissue fluids that are mobilised are virtually electrolyte solutions, protein replacement takes longer.

XX.3 **FTFFF**

A The monosynaptic reflex is not an all-or-none response.

C There is usually (as at the neuromuscular junction) a large safety margin to transmission, but the answer is *false* because there is no logical connection between the stem and the branch: all-or-none is all-or-none whether or not all receptors are needed.

D The grading of activity of skeletal muscle is by recruitment of fibres; each fibre fires all-or-none.

E There is no connection between all-or-none activity and refractoriness.

XX.4 **TFTFT**

A,B Parathormone increases plasma calcium. Remember plasma phosphate is the inverse of calcium, so both these statements cannot be true because they imply that calcium and phosphate increase together.

D Calmodulin is a regulatory protein of calcium at cellular, not plasma, level.

XX.5 **TTTFF**

D The PaO_2 in the normal neonate is about 80 mmHg (10.7 kPa).

E The ductus constricts soon after birth. Species differ in the length of time it takes for the ductus to become obliterated, but it is probably about 24–48 h in humans.

XX.6   TTTTF

Prostaglandins are a family of compounds found in a wide variety of tissues and having a wide variety of biological actions: to quote from one well known textbook, '... they have a bewildering array of actions...' for which '...it is difficult to find a common theme....' Don't waste time desperately trying to learn which prostaglandin has what effect in which tissue.

A   Eicosanoids are derivatives of arachidonic acid.

XX.7   TFTTT

There is no alternative to just learning a list: some people find mnemonics are helpful.

B   The adrenals are L1–L2.

XX.8   TTFTF

C,E   The two sites are in the aortic arch, supplied by the vagus nerve, and in the carotid body, supplied by the glossopharyngeal.

XX.9   TFFTF

B,C   The uptake of nitrous oxide is perfusion-limited; and of oxygen is diffusion-limited only in severe exercise or if there is a diffusion barrier.

D   Diffusion capacity is increased in exercise because of recruitment and dilatation of pulmonary capillaries.

E   There may well be conditions in which compliance and diffusion capacity are both changed, but compliance does not directly affect diffusion.

XX.10   TTFTF

C,E   These are true, but are not consequences of the shape of the curve: a test of reasoning, not of knowledge.

XX.11   FTTTF

Intercellular communication is one of the growth areas of physiology (and pharmacology). Whole journals are devoted to just restricted aspects of the subject. It is difficult to see why practising clinical anaesthetists should have to learn the burgeoning details of these systems (fascinating though they are, so the corollary is 'don't get sidetracked when there is more important basic knowledge to be learned').

A   G-proteins are intracellular. The connection with the neurotransmitter is via the membrane receptor.

D   This is true, but is a detail: do not worry if you did not know.

E   The acetylcholine receptor at the neuromuscular junction is a ligand-gated channel. You should have known this.

XX.12   FFTTF

B   There will be a reflex tachycardia because of the lowered peripheral resistance and blood pressure. However, cardiac work will be decreased.

C   Overall coronary perfusion is not altered, but regional flow is.

XX.13   TTTFT

B   Continuing treatment will allow the iron stores to build up.

D   Gastrointestinal side-effects are common, though not usually a problem if dosage is increased slowly.

E   Overdose is usually accidental (in children) or suicidal.

XX.14   TTFTT

C   Metoclopramide may reach higher concentrations in breast milk than in plasma.

XX.15   TFTTT

A   Do not worry if this is the only part of this question you marked incorrectly. You cannot expect (or be expected) to know the answers to all the options in all the questions in an MCQ paper.

B   There is no effect on pulmonary vascular resistance.

C,D   Both these effects are secondary to increased sympathetic activity.

XX.16 FTTTF

A   The well-known 'stimulant' properties of alcohol are caused by disinhibition of higher functions.

D   The amount metabolised per hour in an individual is constant, and is not increased at increased plasma concentrations.

E   Alcohol is a poor *food*, but a good source of *energy* (7 kcal/g).

XX.17 TTTTT

The phenothiazines are an important group of drugs, with varied effects and side-effects.

E   The balance of adrenergic blockade and anticholinergic action differs between phenothiazines, which means that some dilate and some constrict the pupil. Chlorpromazine constricts the pupil (miosis).

XX.18 TTTTT

E   Decreased pH in inflamed tissue slows absorption by increasing ionisation.

XX.19 TFFTF

A   Although the action of vecuronium wears off because of redistribution, it is also metabolised.

C   This was the reason given for the tachycardia caused by pancuronium.

E   This is a difficult one. You might prefer to use atracurium, but vecuronium is not contraindicated in renal failure.

XX.20 TFFTT

B   Naloxone is N-allyl *oxymorphone*; the allyl group replaces the methyl group of the agonist.

C   Naloxone is not a respiratory stimulant unless the subject has been given opioids.

XX.21 TTTTT

These responses occur in about 10% of patients receiving both drugs and are probably because of interference with metabolism. Pethidine overdose causes similar symptoms.

A   Hypertension can also occur.

XX.22 TFFTT

Increasingly, patients with AIDS will require our services, in theatre and intensive care. Most of them will be taking, or will have taken, zidovudine.

B   There is no injectable form of zidovudine.

C   Almost half the patients will have a problem with marrow depression.

E   Aspirin inhibits glucuronyl transferase reactions, the route of inactivation of zidovudine.

XX.23 TTFFT

C   Any fibrinolytic drug can cause bleeding, whether or not there is thromboembolic disease.

D   Streptokinase is given in large doses because much of it is mopped up by circulating antibody. Almost everybody will have had a streptococcal infection at some time, and allergic (even anaphylactic) reactions are possible in anybody.

XX.24 FTFFT

A   The geometric mean is the logarithmic mean. The so-called logarithmic transformation is a way of allowing the application of statistics based on the normal distribution to be applied to certain skewed data.

C   This is inference in the wrong direction. The population mean has a 95% likelihood of being within the 95% confidence interval of the sample mean.

D   Bias is a more complex matter than can be determined simply by looking at distributions.

E   By convention a large sample is over 100, when the t-distribution differs little from the normal distribution. The z-ratio can then be used instead of the t test. This is small print: well done if you were correct; do not worry if you did not know; be more careful in the actual examination if you guessed that z-ratio sounded like nonsense and so guessed false.

XX.25 FTTFT

A   The mass spectrometer is so named because the behaviour of compounds within it, and hence their measurement, depends on their atomic masses.

D   In anaesthesia, the most common use is in the measurement of carbon dioxide, oxygen and nitrous oxide, but the mass spectrometer can detect more complex molecules as well, provided they can be introduced into the instrument in the gaseous phase.

XX.26   TFTTT
- **B**   The frequency of alternating current in Britain is 50 Hz.
- **C**   The quoted voltage of 240 is the average voltage of alternating current in Britain (technically the *root mean square* voltage).
- **D**   Ohm's law is more usually expressed algebraically as $V = IR$.
- **E**   Impedance is a sort of composite resistance, measured in ohms, and is important in electrical safety (we talk of skin impedance rather than skin resistance). It is also important in the matching of electrical equipment and hence the fidelity of electrical recording.

XX.27   TTTFF
- **D**   Internally, usually 50 joules maximum.
- **E**   Energy is synchronised with the R wave.

XX.28   TFTTT
- **B**   Entonox, a mixture of gases, cannot have a saturated vapour pressure.
- **C**   Below $-5.5°C$ at cylinder pressure of 51 bar, separation may occur. The liquid phase will be 80% nitrous oxide, 20% O_2. Separation does not occur until $-30°C$ at the pipeline pressure of 4 bar.
- **D,E** Yes: these two branches were easy.

XX.29   TTFTT
- **A**   Henry's law only applies at a given temperature.
- **B,C** Surface tension and solubility are unrelated, but there is a grain of truth in the connection: when a liquid boils its surface tension becomes zero, and nor can it dissolve another gas. This is a case of 'a little learning is a dangerous thing'.
- **D,E** Full definitions of these physical constants were 'in the syllabus' of the old Primary, but only passing acquaintance is now necessary. The Bunsen is the one in physical tables; the Ostwald is the more useful to the physiologist.

XX.30   TFTFF
- **B**   A substance cannot be liquefied at its critical temperature; its latent heat of vaporisation is then zero.
- **D**   Latent heat of vaporisation has nothing to do with freezing.
- **E**   If the latent heat of vaporisation was zero at the boiling point, there would be no need to continue to supply energy once a liquid had started to boil, which is obviously untrue — except at the critical temperature.

Index

Questions are listed under broad headings only. There is some overlap between categories; no question is listed more than once. Roman numerals indicate the number of the paper, and the Arabic number that follows is the number of the question on the paper.

Physiology

Pharmacology

Measurement

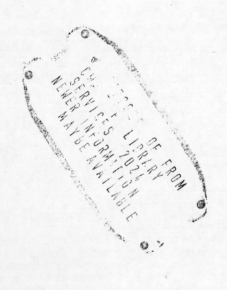